PR
Dr RASHMI SHETTY

'I have known Dr Rashmi for some time now. She treated my skin after a few doctors couldn't figure out what was going on. She is someone who knows what she's doing and her results speak for her work. I trust her judgement and knowledge on skin implicitly.'

Shilpa Shetty Kundra, actor

'I have been associated with Dr Shetty for a couple of years now. Not only is she a great doctor but a superb human being too. She has helped me immensely in some issues that I had seen many doctors for and got no results from. This book will definitely provide all the secrets to what makes her so beautiful too. Lots of love and more success.'

Sania Mirza, Tennis player

'There's always extra pressure when it comes to being in the limelight. Not to mention just being a woman who will inevitably go through life's processes. We all want to look and feel young. So having Dr Rashmi Shetty to look after my skin has been a blessing. With all the travelling, work, and make up I have to wear, I only trust her to make sure my skin is always looking flawless. Thank you Dr Shetty.'

Nargis Fakhri, actor

'Ever since I've understood the meaning of beauty and skincare, I have always been using natural products, including home remedies. But given the industry I am working in, it leaves me exposed to sun, heat, dust, harsh lights etc. So I need a professional hand who will not just help me take care but also enhance the health of my skin and hair. And for this I rely only on Dr Rashmi, who is not only super proficient, her treatment method is very mild and never harsh or strong.'

Yami Gautam, actor

'Dr Rashmi makes you look amazing with her amazing tips and techniques and makes you feel amazing with her lovely, warm, and affable personality—it's a great combination!'

Shruti Hassan, actor

'Meeting Dr Shetty was wonderful. A cosmetic physician who has beautifully blended modern approach to the age-old kitchen beauty tips. The book has interesting and useful information. Grab your copy now!'

Sarika and Akshara, mother-daughter actor duo

'If my hair is good, if my skin is good, it is because of a disciplined lifestyle and Dr Rashmi Shetty.'

Akkineni Nagarjuna, actor

'I trust my directors for the roles I play, and I trust Dr Rashmi Shetty for the role she plays as my hair and skin consultant. My shoot schedules are demanding— be it the harsh lights or pollution outdoors—leaving my skin and hair stressed. Dr Rashmi Shetty's personalized care and right treatment gives me the confidence to take on any challenge. Kudos to Dr Rashmi for this informative book.'

Suriya, actor

'All of us have DNA in our genetics for skin and hair. Dr Rashmi Shetty makes sure you can beautifully flaunt it.'

Rana Daggubati, actor

'In this day and age of confusion, how should one look fresh and happy? I had this question too before I met Dr Rashmi Shetty. Post that, there was no looking back as I knew I will be taken care of.'

Jackky Bhagnani, actor

'Congratulations Dr Rashmi. After years of practice and research, it would be a delight to read *Age Erase*. Wish you the very best with this book.'

Dino Morea, actor

'I first met Dr Shetty at an event I was hosting and I automatically assumed she was the glamorous actress from Hyderabad we were waiting for. We have been friends since then and it's easy to see how much she loves the world of beauty and perfection. Much sought after by corporates for her new-age techniques combined with her knowledge of how to stay beautiful, she travels the world and embodies the essence of a superwoman for me. Which is why I'm really looking forward to her book. She's Doc on call.'

Mini Mathur, Indian TV host, actress, and model

'Dr Shetty is a specialist who I would like to cherish forever. She is a dear friend and undoubtedly an excellent doctor. I met her as my dance student but soon realized the amazing skills she has and since then I only go to her for my skin and hair treatments. I feel fortunate to have a doctor like her who helps me in all possible treatments. Now with a book under her belt, the world will know how amazing her work is. I want to thank her for being there for me and wish her all the best.'

Sandip Soparkar, Latin dance diva and guru

'As an actor and a bodybuilder, I have always found it very hard to keep my skin in optimum condition due to the extreme nature of my two occupations. However, when Dr Rashmi Shetty began treating me, that changed very quickly! Her expertise and knowledge are so rare and I can truly say she surely holds the secret to perfect skin and eternal youth in her capable hands!'

Sahil Khan, actor and bodybuilder

'At Dr Rashmi Shetty's Ra Clinic, I discovered that it was possible to bring out the best of my features while still looking like my natural self. The best part is that Rashmi combines her understanding of aesthetics and psychology while enhancing her client's looks.'

Gajra Kottary, author and scriptwriter, *Balika Vadhu*

'Dr Shetty is a very non-commercial cosmetologist. She tells you what you need (i.e. if you need anything done) and doesn't try to push treatments just to make a buck. I can spend hours with her just chatting as she keeps herself updated with the latest technology available in the market.'

Upasna Kamineni, vice president Apollo Philanthropy and managing director Apollo Life

'One of the few doctors I know who define their "work" as "worship". Best wishes and success always.'

Major (retd.) Sukriti Shuklla, VP-Corporate HR, BDMC Group

'What I love about Dr Rashmi is that she is extremely knowledgeable and is constantly updating herself with the latest in skincare! She has given me a holistic perspective on my skincare regime that was both preventative and proactive.'

Priya Anand, actor

'Dr Rashmi changed the way I look at myself. She pampers skin like no one else.'

Manasi Scott, singer, songwriter, actor

'We live in times where most people—no matter how young or old, famous or not—worry about appearances and have low self-esteem because of it. Dr Rashmi's expertise, insight, and enthusiasm to bring back one's confidence is truly amazing. She breathes life and hope into everything she touches! To me personally, she is a dear friend as well.'

Amala Akkineni, actor and animal activist

'My skin and hair have never looked better. What Dr Rashmi does is magic. She is not like the other doctors

(I've been to the best around the world) who just want to "fix" your face or skin. She cares for you on the whole. Dr Rashmi is an artist.'

Lakshmi Manchu, Hollywood/Indian actor-producer

'Dr Rashmi Shetty's extensive knowledge in cosmetology, coupled with her aesthetic vision and passion for her discipline, is what's making me look forward to her very first book, *Age Erase*. After all, as Dr Shetty always points out, beauty is much deeper than skin.'

Chandi Parera, actress, Sri Lanka

'A woman with a "Midas touch". Rashmi and I go back a long way. I found a beautiful friend and a human being in a doctor who very sincerely takes care of her clients. Thank you so much for always making me look my best.'

Shilpi Sharma, actor, DJ

'I never felt that I was under treatment. Rather, the lovely care made me feel like I was pampered with utmost care. Well, this is something which is unique to her as her spa-like clinic ends up giving you the perfect result as well.'

Amla Paul, actor

'Rashmi has a very holistic approach to skincare. She makes sure to give you solutions for the long run which are easy to follow and maintain. I bless the day I met her.'

Tamannaah Bhatia, actor

'Dr Rashmi is not only a doctor to me but has been a friend for long. Whenever I have skin related issues, the person I speak to is her. I trust her completely with my face.'

Aamir Ali, film and TV actor

'There is no problem or pimple too big for Dr Rashmi Shetty and a few of her magical touches. She is one of the most positive and happy people I have met. She's fabulous with skin and knows it inside out.'

Adha Khan, actor

'Thank you, doctor. You fixed me. In the Coldplay kind of way.'

Samantha Ruth Prabhu, actress

'Rashmi is an angel in my life. I was fighting my skin pigmentation and thankfully met her at the right time. It's been a changed world ever since I walked into Rashmi's clinic. She has been a wonderful friend and not just a great doctor. I am enjoying my womanhood thanks to her. I think of her every time I a complemented for the glow on my face.'

Suguna Srikrishnan, homemaker

'Dr Rashmi Shetty, with her well-equipped knowledge of skin, studies you as a person and gives you that confidence which everyone woman needs. I am glad I gave myself to her at this early age. I trust her and love her from the bottom of my heart.'

Neetu Chandra, film and theatre actor, martial arts expert, Kathak dancer

'What kept me from going to aesthetic doctors was my apprehension for anything invasive and drastic. But when I met Dr Rashmi Shetty, she just fixed me with the least that there can be. Little things like eating right, sleeping well, keeping the scalp clean, and following a skincare regime is all what it took to keep me looking beautiful even on the most stressful days.'

Anita Dongre, designer

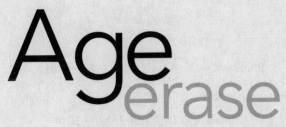

Age erase

YOUR ULTIMATE BEAUTY BIBLE TO AGEING GRACEFULLY

DR RASHMI SHETTY

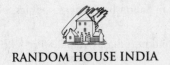

RANDOM HOUSE INDIA

Published by Random House India in 2014
1

Copyright © Dr Rashmi Shetty 2014

Random House Publishers India Private Limited
7th Floor, Infinity Tower C, DLF Cyber City
Gurgaon–122 002
Haryana, India

Random House Group Limited
20 Vauxhall Bridge Road
London SW1V 2SA
United Kingdom

978 81 8400 516 5

Any advice in terms of supplements, generic ingredients of
cosmeceuticals, or any mention of a trade name in the book
should be taken only upon your doctor's recommendation.

Typeset in Sabon by Saanvi Graphics, Noida

Printed and bound in India by Replika Press Private Limited

To the two most beautiful ladies in my life—

my mom who taught me the importance of beauty and presentation in everything I do

and my daughter who is the 'every woman in my life'.

If not for them, I wouldn't have achieved what I have today.

CONTENTS

Part I

ALL ABOUT SKIN

Part II

CHEAT THE CLOCK

INTRODUCTION

'A THING OF BEAUTY is a joy forever', said the romantic poet John Keats. Whether it is a beautiful structure, a painting, a flower, or a face, it ultimately brings joy to your heart. We all want to look beautiful but we somehow think it is vain to acknowledge it or give it its due importance.

I always wanted to be involved in the aesthetic branch of medicine. But while I was in medical school, aesthetic work was considered the domain of plastic surgeons and not physicians or dermatologists. Then came in innovation in the form of Botox, various fillers, and equipments that made aesthetic enhancement and maintaining a youthful face and body an office or a day-care procedure. There was so much that could be achieved with just the right portion in a pot! So I decided to specialize in the aesthetic and cosmetic part of skincare and anti-ageing. Soon, there I was—completely loving my work and what I could do with it, and smiling to myself knowing how many lives I could touch with my work.

I started my practice 13 years ago in a polyclinic which Dr Meera Agarwal, the famous gynaecologist, had directed me to. I still remember when I came back from England wanting to have an exclusive cosmetic practice, none of the hospitals had even a department for it whereas today most hospitals have a floor dedicated to it. I then met some of my senior doctors from Lilavati Hospital where I was working as a resident and told them all about my specialization and by and by my practice grew through word of mouth.

When my juniors at various teaching workshops and the conferences I attend ask me how I reached where I am today, I always have the same story to tell them.

There is no magic! I sat there in my polyclinic for 3 long months without any patients. Then the first one trickled and then another, till I was thrown out one day as I was eating into all other doctors' time. The rest as they say is history. I was also was a part of Breach Candy Hospital's private clinics but I realized in a year that this branch of medicine required a much more private setting and so I set up my own space—Ra Skin 'n' Aesthetics in Mumbai and REVA Health and Skin in Hyderabad. Today these are busy practices where I work from 10 am to 8 pm with lunch on the go. On the academic front, I am on the scientific advisory boards of various world forums, give lectures around the world, and I am a key opinion leader for various cosmeceutical and medical-device firms, interacting with global thought leaders.

By no stretch of imagination have I ever perceived my work as being medically insignificant as compared to other medical practitioners. Just as a psychiatrist's patient should ideally emerge from the course of treatment with a whole new positive perspective on life—which in turn becomes a self-fulfilling prophecy for him/her—an aesthetician too has the capability to turn around a human being's quality of life. When I was a resident at the Bangalore hospital under my plastic surgery boss Dr K.S. Shekar, we used to operate on a lot of cleft lip and palate patients. We were a part of 'Smile Train'—a worldwide programme to operate all children with cleft lips free of cost. The joy it brought to them and their parents was divine. Later when they came in for follow-ups, though functionally they looked good, the remnant signs were there—the scar, the unsmooth lip, the slight defect of the shape of the nose. I'd listen to them talk about how they wished they could have no signs of their defects at all. That was my defining moment! I instantly knew I wanted to get into appearance medicine—whatever it takes to give a great finishing.

In my debut book on beauty, I intend to bring out the best of what I have learnt through my medical graduation from AIMS in Bellur, Karnataka, further studies in Cosmetic Dermatology from Chester, UK, and most of all from my 12 years of exclusive practice in aesthetic medicine and anti-ageing at my clinics in Mumbai and Hyderabad. In these years, I have treated a gamut of patients—from homemakers to jet-setting business heads, little teen daughters of my patients (who I keep driving away so nature can take its course) and even women at 70. I have worked on supermodels and actors from Bollywood and Tollywood, my own doctor friends from all specialities and their children, and women and men of all ethnicity as I conduct hands-on teaching courses at various dermatologic and plastic surgery forums across India, Europe, USA, and the Far East. This, and my academic association with scientific committees and advisory boards of Anti-ageing Medicine World Congress (AMWC) and Anti-ageing Medicine European Congress(AMEC), keeps me up-to-date with the absolute latest in the field of aesthetic dermatology.

Essentially, I've realized that the concerns, wants, and needs of women and men are by and large consistent all over the world. We all want to look young and beautiful and the pressure to maintain a youthful self becomes a constant stress factor in our lives. We also know how our body language becomes a tool for others to judge us. The other day I was listening to a TED talk and was intrigued by American psychologist Amy Cuddy's talk on how our body language affects our own behaviour and influences our mind. I believe likewise. Have you noticed how your mood and behaviour is on a day when you look in the mirror and know you look super?

This book is therefore my mission as well as my vision to bring beauty back to the centre stage of people's lives, not as a weapon, but as a tool to carve out a happier life first for oneself and then for all those around.

WHY THIS BOOK?

I'VE WRITTEN THIS BOOK primarily because:

- A majority of people need a guiding hand to understand their 'skin crisis' and the vast variety of treatments and products available today.
- Most people are shy of acknowledging that they now feel like taking care of their skin.
- The mystery of finding the right doctor is daunting.
- The men out there cringe and wonder how they'll ever walk into a skin clinic.
- When you finally do go to a doctor, your forget most of your questions in the limited time you have with the doctor.
- And then you find yourself holding back from asking for information thinking you might be pressured into signing up for treatments you are not keen on.
- No book has brought together so many wonderful experts giving you home care, nutrition, exercise,

and make up tips in one place for you to sink your teeth into.

So why should one take care of one's skin at all when half of us believe that it is genetically pre-determined and the other half believes that 'ageing gracefully' is just letting yourself age without any active intervention? Here's why.

We need to understand that 50 percent of what we are is what we are born with. The other 50 percent depends on how we take care of what we have. In today's times, with all the processed food, pollution, stress, multitasking, all sorts of electronic signals, extreme diets to keep up with new social norms of wanting the body of a 20-year-old at 50 etc., personal care becomes all the more challenging. Our parents were exposed to none of this, so naturally they had better skin and aged more gracefully with very less or no effort at all. But today, you can't afford to go by what they did or didn't. Our urban and sedentary lifestyles demand that we workout and eat right if we want to stay healthy and beautiful.

Now analyse this—the pretty and the not-so-pretty, the handsome and the not-so-handsome, the bold and the beautiful—all will inevitably age. It is a process that begins with our birth and will stay with us like an unwanted but devoted companion. Our philosophy in accepting its presence and dealing with its effects will most likely be erratic.

Small children want to hurry the process of growing up so they can be 'big and strong like daddy' and 'wear mamma's lipstick and blush-on'; teenagers can't wait to get out of school and join college and get their driving licenses. Boys can't wait to be shaving like papa and girls rush to get their first facial and eyebrows threaded. But then comes the first pimple that scares you and from there on, your worries begin. Yet the heady elixir of sheer youth usually makes up for it and worries often cease, despite the pimple!

Then life takes over, and soon you are in the middle of a whirlwind of romance, jobs, marriage, parenthood, finances, stress, strain, and before you know it, you look into the mirror and see that you have aged. It could be a single grey hair or an almost cute wrinkle or even the fact that the neighbour's kid called you 'uncle' or 'aunt'. And unintentionally, you soon wistfully wish for the time when you were younger, had more time to correct the wrong, and you want to now turn back the clock.

Ageing we are and age we will. What we can do however, is try to walk the journey gracefully and beautifully. Women come to see me purely for beauty and nobody can convince me otherwise. They may say I don't like a fold or a hollow, I don't like a blemish, I don't like a dark spot, but what they are trying to tell or wanting is to be more beautiful. Mind you, a lot of my patients are models and movie stars who are already beautiful! As Dr Arthur Swift, an expert plastic surgeon from Montreal, Canada, mentioned in one of his talks, 'American studies looked at women between the age of 20 and 60 and asked them that what is the No. 1 reason for you to go and see a plastic surgeon and the No. 1 answer was to be more beautiful. That didn't make sense because there were women amongst that group who were already absolutely stunning and models but they still wanted to be more beautiful. So women are beauty seekers. Men on the other hand want to be more virile or youthful.' Or 'youthful contenders' as Dr Swift calls them.

Ageing can mean different things to different people and at different stages. Growing from an awkward teen to a pretty 20 something to a beautiful 30-year-old and then a serene, confident 40-year-old might be termed as pleasant. Then, as time battles age, the not so pleasant changes begin to manifest more apparently. But not anymore. With scientific innovation in skincare, you have all the information at your disposal to look and feel your best—whether it's regular skincare, or advanced medical procedures.

What you see in your mirror not only makes an impression on the world but also on you, your mood, efficiency, and your attitude. So read on to know the whats, whys, and hows of ageing, where and why the changes occur, how simple and basic dos and don'ts can make a difference, and what chances the anti-ageing products and treatments offer.

Age Erase is a culmination of all of my 13 years of speciality practice and what I learnt before that, compressed into an easy-to-read informative format for you to know at your own pace and place. So read on and see how you can put your best face forward.

HOW TO USE THIS BOOK?

FOR ANYONE WHO WANTS to age gracefully, this book will tell you how to do just that. But before you embark on this journey with me, my one piece of advice to you would be to read it all—from page 1 to the very end—and not just selective sections. For example, if you are 40-years-old and looking for something that makes you look your best, it's not enough for you to read just that section. You'd benefit immensely from sections like care for the lips and eyes, the right nutrition and skin regimen, and many more. So do not restrict yourself and be open to exploring a lot more as you read along.

Right from important notes and do-it-yourself tips to medical advice and even cures for men, this book will have it all. But mostly, the information in the book is gender inclusive and works for both sexes. The book is divided into two parts, with seven chapters in each part.

PART I: All About Skin, will answer all your basic questions about skin.

- ❖ Chapter 1, Know Your Skin, talks about the layers that make up the skin, it's important functions and classifications, the five vital signs of healthy skin and the role our DNA plays in how our skin is, looks, and feels.
- ❖ Chapter 2 talks about the major skin issues that cause stress like open pores, adult acne, pigmentation, etc.
- ❖ Chapter 3 talks about how hormones like oestrogen, progesterone, thyroid hormones etc. affect our skin and hair.
- ❖ Chapter 4 highlights the most common skincare emergencies like tan burns and itchy skin.
- ❖ Chapter 5 shows you why good sleep is crucial to beautiful skin.
- ❖ Chapter 6 talks about the effects the changing weather—summer, monsoon, winter—has on our skin.
- ❖ Part I ends with Chapter 7 on bridal, travel, and festival skincare.

Part II, Cheat the Clock, will guide you through tried and tested beauty fundas to help you age beautifully.

- ❖ Chapter 8 is an in-depth chapter on the basic skin-care essentials that every individual must own.
- ❖ Chapter 9 focuses on necessary nutrients required to keep the hair and skin in top shape.

❖ Chapter 10 decodes the components of your skincare regime.

❖ Chapter 11 essentially talks about the process of ageing, photoageing and sun protection, calculating one's skin age and the importance of matching it with the right skincare. From your teens to your 60s and beyond, skincare for all age groups is covered. Here I will also be talking about taking special care of the eyes, lips, neck and chest, hands and body, and nutrients for skin and hair.

❖ Chapter 12 lists down anti-ageing treatments that one could go for and certain age aggressors that one needs to be careful of.

❖ Chapter 13 will tell you how to read cosmetic labels and ingredients like an expert. There is also a section on male grooming specifics.

❖ Chapter 14, the final chapter, is on goodies for great skincare and includes information on anti-ageing workouts, facial massages, food recipes, and home remedies. For this chapter, I have taken the advice of certain experts in the fields of fitness, nutrition, and naturopathy because that is not my area of expertise and I do not wish to dole out wrong information to my readers. I hope all of you will benefit from their advice and put it to great use. Thank you to all the experts who have contributed to my book, for taking out time from your busy schedules to help us better understand the importance of right nutrition and diet as we age, how fitness is important to help us retain our youthful self, and how simple home remedies can make so much of a difference.

Age Erase is not just about ageing, lines, or pigmentation spots. It's about changes you may notice in your skin and the transformations that it goes through as you transition from one decade to another. This book looks at ageing as a process and aims to help you age gracefully. So go ahead and take that first step to eternal youth!

Part I
All About Skin

CHAPTER 1

KNOW YOUR SKIN

THANK GOD FOR OUR SKIN! Like a wrapper protects a candy bar, the skin acts as the wrapper for our body. So imagine walking around without our wrapper. With all our muscles, nerves, internal organs visible, how freaky it would be! Never mind how smooth or what colour it is, keeping your skin healthy is important.

Let me start by telling you a bit about skin, its various structures and functions, and some interesting facts related to it.

It is the largest and one of the most dynamic organs in the body

The skin is also most exposed to the outside, making it vulnerable to ambient humidity, pollution, temperature, sun etc. Therefore, it is necessary to take constant account of your surroundings and notice what it is doing to your skin. Some surroundings may leave you with a short-term and quickly reversible effect like dryness while some may leave you with long-term damage which may take much longer to undo—like the harmful rays of the sun.

It is elastic to a certain extent and has the tendency to adapt to the changes in your body size as you put on and lose body mass—like muscle, fat, or pregnancy weight

Just imagine if the skin on your abdomen never shrunk back after pregnancy! Or it never went back to wrapping your newly acquired muscular body. But there is only so much that the skin can handle. So like any other expandable thing, it reaches a breaking point and if the elastin breaks up and the collagen gets too pulled, you end up getting stretch marks. At times there may be skin excess that may have to be surgically removed but by and large if you are patient for 2 to 3 months, the skin shrinks back.

70 percent of the skin is water

There you go! Now you know why every skincare article that you ever read on the Internet or in a magazine tells you to drink a minimum of 8 glasses of water every day to keep the skin hydrated. However, I do not insist on the number. It is important that you hydrate well. Whether with water, tender coconut water, buttermilk, vegetable juice, soup—I leave it to you. If you lose water a lot during the day, be it through perspiration or staying in the air conditioning for too long. When you are dehydrated, it will show on your skin and your system will go haywire—your mouth will feel parched, your lips will turn dry, the colour of your urine will become darker, and your skin will feel dull and lifeless.

25 percent is protein

Protein is not only important for people on a special weight loss or muscle building programme but for all of us—young or old. Protein is your building block. It helps build and repair pretty much every tissue of your body, including your hair and nails. So it is very important that you make protein a good part of your natural daily diet. Any kind of supplements should be taken under expert advice only.

5 percent is fats and minerals

Time and again I have seen that the first thing a person on a weight loss spree does is stop the intake of rice and oil. This is a bad idea. Yes, anything in excess is harmful for the body, but totally cutting out any one food component is no good either. You need at least 2 spoons of any form of oil, be it coconut, olive, rice bran, or ghee in your daily food plan. If not, it tells on your skin, hair, and the general health of your organs. There are certain important micronutrients like fat-soluble vitamins that may not get absorbed at all. So not only does your skin need moisturizing from the outside, it also needs it from the inside, and definitely more so if you are 30 plus. And when you reach your 50s, the subcutaneous fat or the fat beneath your skin starts thinning to a point that a specific type of eczema called asteatotic eczema develops. It is characterized by itching and severe dryness of skin, especially on the shin and lower extremities. This scratching leads to wounds.

Common terms associated with skin

NMF: You have often seen the letters NMF written on the lotions you buy. NMF stands for Natural Moisturising Factor. NMFs make up an expansive group of ingredients that include amino acids, ceramides, hyaluronic acid, cholesterol, fatty acids, triglycerides, phospholipids, glycosphingolipids, urea, linoleic acid, glycosaminoglycans, glycerin, mucopolysaccharides, and sodium PCA (pyrrolidone carboxylic acid). The creams that have urea, lactate, or any of the ingredients mentioned above also add to the NMF on your skin. They help stabilize and maintain this complex intercellular-skin matrix. Using moisturizers of any kind that contain NMFs allows your skin to do its job of repairing and regenerating itself without the impedances brought on when skin is suffering from dryness, environmental distress, or excess irritation.

Lipids: They are the fats in the skin that give the skin its bounce. The lipids in stratum corneum are found between dead skin layers, which also maintain the hydration factor of the skin. Intercellular lipids have 40–50% ceramides, 20–25% cholesterol, 15–25% fatty acids, and 5–10% cholesterol sulphate. They make 15% of the dry weight of the dead layer. These lipids of the epidermis decide the hydration and the oil content of the skin.

Collagen: Collagen is the most abundant protein in our body, accounting for around 30% of the protein content of the human body. Collagen fibres are soft and flexible, but also strong and inelastic. They make up almost 75% of the dry weight of your skin and comprise the major component of the dermis. There are different types, type 1 being the most abundant collagen in the body.

Elastin: Elastin forms a continuous network throughout the dermis. It maintains the normal configuration of the skin due to its elastic recoiling. It undergoes significant changes upon sun exposure and with age.

Layers of skin

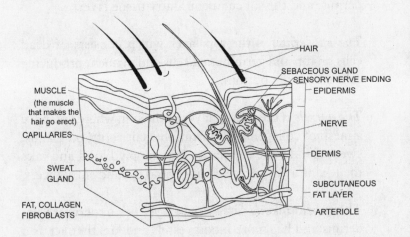

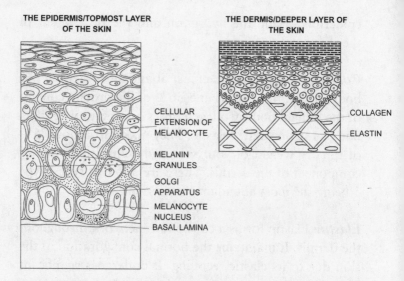

THE EPIDERMIS/TOPMOST LAYER OF THE SKIN

THE DERMIS/DEEPER LAYER OF THE SKIN

CELLULAR EXTENSION OF MELANOCYTE

MELANIN GRANULES

GOLGI APPARATUS

MELANOCYTE NUCLEUS
BASAL LAMINA

COLLAGEN

ELASTIN

Skin by and large has many layers but I am not going into too much detail about it. What you need to know about are the three major layers—the epidermis, the dermis, and the subcutaneous fatty tissue layer.

The epidermis is the top layer which consists of dead cells on top and germinating cells and pigment producing cells etc. at the bottom.

The dermis is the central layer of the skin where you have a mesh of collagen and elastin, the hair roots, oil glands, sweat glands, the capillaries that supply blood and take the toxins away, nerve endings, and ground substance.

The subcutaneous fatty tissue layer lies underneath the dermis and has more blood vessels and fats that act as a cushion to your skin.

Functions of the skin

> ➢ Protection: It acts as a barrier, protecting our body from environmental impact and microorganisms.
> ➢ Regulation: It maintains body temperature through sweat and hair—one of the essentials for a healthy body.
> ➢ Sensation: The network of nerve cells helps us feel through touch, pain, heat, and cold.
> ➢ Excretion and Secretion: Sweat is not just water. It also contains urea and creatinin which act like toxin excretion. Secretions like sebum keeps the skin oil balanced and keep the natural microorganisms of the skin in a healthy state.

Skin as a protective organ

Now you know why you should not scrub off the top dead layer aggressively. Also do not wash your skin too many times or you may one, strip all the natural secretions and two, trigger a feedback from the skin when it is super dry and cause the oil glands to over-secrete. Excessive skin peeling treatments make the skin more vulnerable to damage. Especially avoid those treatments that rip your outer dead skin layer off before you go on a sunny or a beach holiday.

Skin also acts as a barrier against water loss. Trans-epidermal water loss is water that passes from your deeper tissues through the epidermal layer to the surrounding atmosphere via diffusion and evaporation process. The water loss from the skin is affected by the level of humidity, temperature, weather, and your skin's natural moisture content.

This is a continuous process over which we have little control. It can increase due to disruption to the skin barrier due to wounds, scratches, burns, or exposure to harsh surfactants. This leads to extreme dryness of the skin. Disturbance in any layer of the skin causes a loss of water from the skin.

The stratum corneum has 30% water which is associated with elasticity of the outer layer of the skin. The innermost layer of the stratum corneum has the maximum percentage of water that supports the outer layer. The moisture on the outermost layer of the skin is dependent on the ambient humidity.

Thirdly, the skin is your biggest immune guard that keeps you safe from infections. But when you have chapped skin or cuts, you have to be extra careful. This is especially important during the monsoon months when there is higher humidity and more chances of bacteria to grow. So keep your skin clean and dry, yet hydrated as well.

But there is a flip side to this. Since the skin forms a protective barrier, the lotions that you apply play a major role in the kind of protection offered to your skin. You have to choose products from skincare companies that are research-oriented because they use the right vehicles, right version of the actives (key ingredients or ingredients that give you the desired result), and the appropriate molecular size to deliver the ingredients into the skin through the top layer.

Skin as an excretory and secretory organ

The skin helps you sweat out toxins and chemicals. So, when you are at the gym and working out, I would not advise you to repeatedly wipe yourself with a hand towel. You should instead wash your sweat off the skin with water or use a facial mist spray and dab it off with a face tissue. Avoid using any heavy moisturizers or make up or even sunscreens if you are working out indoors.

Also, do not, I stress, *do not* put any skincare products or make up on sweaty skin as it will mix with the toxins already on top and make things worse.

There are 3 units that can cause trouble if blocked. 1. With sweat glands, they are seen as tiny bumps at times beneath your eye, treated best with burning them with radio frequency(or simply by nipping them off under aseptic precautions with the right sized needle) at your doctor's clinic. 2. With sebaceous/oil glands you see them as whiteheads when they are closed with a layer of skin on top; blackheads when they are open and the content gets oxidized when in contact with oxygen in air; acne, when this gets infected, or cysts. The whole unit of oil gland and hair follicle could be affected which is when it is called pilosebaceous cyst or abscess. 3. Only hair follicle blocked and infected, shows up as tiny white pus boils at the base of your hair i.e folliculitis. This could be on any hair bearing part of the skin on your body, scalp, or beard area for men.

Skin as a sense organ and temperature regulator

We all know skin is a sensory organ. How else would we feel the touch of a loved one? Your skin maintains the temperature of your body too. This may make the skin look either pale or flushed depending on the weather or outside environmental conditions.

For example, in winter your skin looks pale because it is trying to regulate the body heat by constricting the blood vessels in the periphery. The opposite happens in summer when you have dilated capillaries to let the heat escape, and more blood flows into the skin. This makes you look flushed and red.

In both cases, you have to ensure that you don't let the extremes happen. So when it is flushed in summer, you have to calm it down with a splash of cold water or with an application of cold calamine. In winter you have to wash it with warm water to keep the circulation going. You can also use little tapping movements over your skin to stimulate it by using the flat inner surface of the full length of your fingers. You can bend down to get blood rushing to the skin or you can try a head or shoulder stand position if you are a yoga enthusiast.

So here you are—your own skin expert!

Classification of skin type (by colour and response to sun)

Skin types can be classified in many ways. But the two classifications that will help you to choose skincare and procedures will be the ones determined by the oil and water content of your skin, and by the colour and response to the sun.

The first step in assessing your skin is washing your face really well at night. Go to bed without putting anything on your face. Avoid having any air-conditioning or heater on; you could leave your fan on though. Then, when you get up in the morning, pat your face all over. Specifically, check your:

- ⚜ T-Zone which is from the centre of your forehead down your nose and chin; and includes the part of cheek next to your nose
- ⚜ C-Zone which is the part of your cheek nearer to the ears and your jawline, temple, and forehead near the hairline

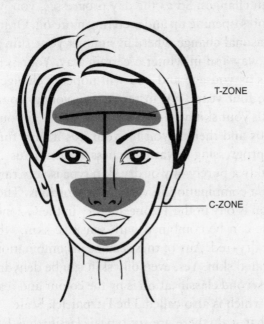

Now see if they feel oily or dry. If the area is greasy, you obviously have oily skin. If it feels crepey (dry) and fine-textured, you are dry skinned. If you feel some areas are dry and some oily, you have a combination skin type.

Some signs that you can look out for

If you have large open pores, then you have oily skin. If the pores are tightly shut, then you have dry skin. If your skin looks red and flushed, you have sensitive skin. If you have flaky and chapped skin or lips, visible fine lines, it is too dry and dehydrated.

However, this does not mean that your skin will remain the same for the rest of your life. It could only be for that day or that moment. You may even notice intra-day skin changes. So as the day progresses, you will see your pores opening up and secreting more oil. Or it could be a seasonal change where in summer your skin feels a certain way and in winter a certain way. Your skin also changes as you age and you will notice a change every three to four years. For instance, as a young woman, in your 20s your skin was oily which turns dry as you reach your 30s and then as you hit your 40s it may turn oily again, progressing towards dryness at menopause.

Frankly a purely oily or dry skin type is very rare. It is usually a combination in various proportions. The most common is oily in the T-zone and dry in the C-zone. Any of these can be combined with sensitive skin, which is usually dry+red. Any of these can be in combination with dehydrated skin. Yes, even oily skin can be dehydrated.

The second classification is by the colour and response to sun which is also called **The Fitzpatrick Scale**.

By that scale there are six types, classified as I, II, III, IV, V, VI. While Caucasians mostly have skin types I and II and Africans type VI, we Indians usually fall under skin type III, IV or V. So here's how you decide what is your skin type:

- ❖ **Type I** Pale white; blonde or red hair; blue eyes; freckles.
  Always burns, never tans.
- ❖ **Type II** White; fair; blonde or red hair; blue, green or hazel eyes.
  Usually burns, tans minimally.
- ❖ **Type III** Creamy white; fair with any hair or eye colour; quite common.
  Sometimes mild burn, tans uniformly.
- ❖ **Type IV** Moderate brown; typical Mediterranean skin tone.
  Rarely burns, always tans well.
- ❖ **Type V** Dark brown; Middle Eastern skin type.
  Very rarely burns, tans very easily.
- ❖ **Type VI** Deeply pigmented; dark brown to black.
  Never burns, tans very easily.

Remember, even if your skin type may not have burning sensation, does not mean that sun rays are not harming your skin. A tan will definitely show up—it might be immediate or delayed.

The glow factor

I know for certain that every one's skin has the potential to glow. It's just a matter of how you look after it that decides how healthy it looks. Some people are blessed with good genes and start off well. All they need is to take a little care of their skin. But sadly, these people sometimes take their skin for granted and come to me in a panicked state when it is far into the damage zone. Some of us are not so blessed and our skin may need correction and constant care.

Then there are the two types of people with extreme attitudes. The first are those who come running the day they hit 20 and ask me endless questions about changes that occur with ageing. They are so sure they need surgery right then and there. Besides turning down most of their requests, I have to calm them down with advice on what they actually need.

The second types are those who let go so badly in the name of 'ageing gracefully'! To me this term means so much more than looking beautiful. It means someone who at their age looks so serene and beautiful that it makes me wish I look half as good as them when I reach their age.

5 signs of healthy skin

If you have good and healthy skin, you find friends complementing you on your glowing skin and asking you about the secret recipe to it. You feel nice, happy, and energetic, and your skin, hair, and nails glow even brighter with confidence. When you don't have great skin, either you ignore it or you work at improving it because you know the negative impact it has on you, your confidence, your mood, relationships, and sometimes even your efficiency.

But getting that healthy glow does not come after following just one step. Most patients come to me and ask for the secret to glowing skin as if there's a bulb in them that I can turn on. Like I said before, your outside, i.e. your skin and how it looks, affects your insides, your mood, and your health. And what you put inside—your nutrition—shows on the outside.

So before we move ahead, let's first talk about how a healthy, beautiful skin should look and feel.

#1 *Even skin tone:* Your skin should have a consistent colour no matter what your complexion is. It does not matter if you are fair, dusky, or dark; the evenness of skin tone is what makes you look attractive. Little shadows are natural to Indian skin tone. But for it to look attractive, the colour graduation has to be seamless, blending with the rest of your facial skin colour.

#2 *Well hydrated:* You know skin has enough moisture when it feels supple to the touch. Another way of knowing whether your skin is well hydrated is when your skin bounces back as you press and release it. You know then that the lipid barrier is well preserved, causing minimal transepidermal water loss.

#3 *Smooth texture:* Healthy skin looks smooth and feels smooth. If you look closely in the mirror, you will notice a uniform layout of your pores, and tiny peaks around your hair follicles (yes, our face does have a very fine layer of hair, almost invisible to the naked eye). The pores are small, tight, and feel smooth to touch.

 # 4 *Reflects light:* Your skin is neither too dry or chapped nor too oily. The pores are closed. This makes the light that hits your face travel back in a straight line instead of scattering it, so that a person looking at you sees your skin shine and glow.

#5 *Normal sensations:* When your skin is healthy, you will not feel any irregular sensations like stretching, burning, or itching.

Is there a way to guess how you may age?

Stand with a hand mirror in your hand and look at your reflection in the mirror, with your hair tied up. Bend forward to look at your face more closely and that's how you will look 5 years later. Bend backwards or lay down with the mirror on top and that's how you looked 5 years ago. You have the potential to get back to how you looked 5 years ago with right care and intervention.

Your skin DNA

Recently there has been a lot of hype about customizing one's skincare products as per the DNA analyses of the skin. Yes, sure science has gotten this specific. But do we really need it? First, let me tell you that despite all the testing that's being done, all that research has told you is whether your skin needs anti dry/anti lines/anti free radicals/anti redness/anti pigment ingredients more in your skincare creams or not. But don't we already know most of it?

Remember remarks like, 'Look at your mom-in-law to see how your wife will age'. Just look at your parents and siblings and you'll know what elements of ageing you should focus on most.

One of my actor patients was once telling me, 'Doctor, my special skill is that I can cry onstage or when a shot demands it. Or I can let a tear drop slowly from my eye if I'm shooting a sad scene. Also, I can grow a pimple in real time basis when stressed.' Likewise, we all know how we react to stress, certain food substances, menstrual cycles, and dust in a specific way.

Supposing both you and your friend suffer from the same skin problem, say pigmentation. Even though you may end up buying the same skin product, you will notice that a particular product may give her better results while your skin will show no signs of improvement. The answer to this must lie deeper in the skin.

Your cells are coded in such a way that they react to different actives in different ways even if the skin issue is the same. This is where your doctor's experience counts in looking at your history and signs that your skin gives out—like pigmentation on stress areas like say body folds and elbows/knees or the pattern of skin reacting during cycles and seasonal changes—and then identifying and changing the ingredients. So what works for you may not work for your friend and you must go to an expert for the right opinion.

The role genes play in your hair and skin

- ❖ Your skin's genetic tendency to get acne
- ❖ How your skin will age in terms of wrinkles, sagging, neck ageing
- ❖ How your hair will change with age in terms of the texture, density and overall health
- ❖ How and when you'll bald
- ❖ When you may start greying
- ❖ When you may enter menopause

- How your skin forms scars
- How your skin will pigment
- How your skin will react to the sun or other external factors
- How fast oxidation will damage your skin
- How you will heal from an injury to your skin
- How your skin, hair, and nails will respond to any treatments or products applied to them

By putting the two together, you know what to remember in your skincare routine and what to stress on when you seek professional help towards ageing gracefully.

Other important skincare terms

Transepidermal water loss: Skin acts as a major barrier against transepidermal water loss. Transepidermal water loss is water that passes from inside your body through the epidermal layer to the surrounding atmosphere via diffusion and evaporation process. The water loss from the skin is affected by the level of humidity, temperature, season, and your skin's natural moisture content. This is a continuous process over which we have little control. It can increase due to disruption to the skin barrier due to wounds, scratches, burns, and exposure to harsh surfactants. This leads to extreme dryness. Disturbance in any layer of the skin causes this loss of water from the skin.

Stratum corneum has 30% water which is associated with elasticity of the outer layer of the skin. The innermost layer of stratum corneum has the maximum percent of water that supports the outer layer. The moisture on the outermost layer of the skin is dependent on the ambient humidity.

Skin pH: pH is the measurement of acidity. But what does that mean in the context of your skin? It means the acid mantle over your skin, which acts as a barrier and prevents infections. This acid mantle is also important in controlling the enzyme activity on the skin and in skin renewal. pH is measured from 1 upwards, with 1 being highly acidic and 14 being highly alkaline. A pH of 7 is neutral. A pH between 1 and 6 is acidic and between 7 and 14 is alkaline. The optimal pH of our skin is 5.5. The layer of sweat and sebum together make the acid mantle. In fact the condition of the pH on your skin is dependent on internal factors like natural moisture, oil glands, sweat, genetic predisposition and age. Externally, skin's pH balance can become affected by harsh soaps, astringent, medication, face wash, and cosmetics.

Using astringent soap or face wash removes the acid mantle and can leave your skin vulnerable to problems like acne, contact dermatitis, fungal and bacterial infections.

Free Radicals: Free radicals are atoms or groups of atoms with unpaired number of electrons that are formed when oxygen interacts with certain molecules. Oxidation is a very natural process that happens during normal cellular functions.

Now these unpaired electrons literally go on a rampage trying to attach to electrons from other molecules. So these highly reactive radicals react with important cellular components such as DNA or the cell membrane and damage them. After reacting with a free radical, the cells generally function poorly or die. Once free radicals react with the cellular DNA, they cause mutation and abnormality which then shows up on various organs including skin. Since 1956 doctors and scientists have agreed that free radicals are one of the major causes of premature ageing of skin.

External toxins like UV rays, pollution, and cigarette smoke are the biggest reasons why free radicals are produced in our bodies. This oxidative stress on the skin cells can be prevented by supporting your skin with antioxidants. You need to protect skin by both taking antioxidant supplements and eating antioxidant rich foods and applying creams and lotions with added antioxidant actives.

Enzymes: Enzymes are chemicals that speed up the rate of chemical reactions without being consumed in the reaction themselves. Our skin enzymes have two main uses: One for exfoliation and the other as an anti-inflammatory. In fact, enzymes derived from fruits are effective exfoliants and are often gentler than other methods like scrubs and microdermabrasion.

The enzymes work by specifically breaking down the keratin protein or the top dead layer, revealing the newer, smoother skin below. They are able to digest keratin protein and stratum corneum, thus strengthening healthy skin with natural antioxidant vitamins as they exfoliate.

In skincare, the most popular and commonly used exfoliating enzymes are derived from pineapple, papaya and pumpkin. Pineapple contains the strongest of the three enzymes called bromelain. Papaya contains the enzyme papain, and pumpkin is rich in the enzyme protease. The enzymes in these fruits are so potent that you can actually mash them up and apply on your face and get supple skin in a few minutes. The antioxidants that are added to the skin as these enzymes work are vitamin A from pumpkin's protease, and vitamin C from pineapple's bromelain and papaya's papain. Other fruits that have skin smoothing enzymes include grapes, strawberries, pomegranate, and cherries.

These enzymes function as a scavenger of free radicals and protect the skin against oxidative damage. Simply put, enzymes can protect against damage from the sun, environmental pollutants, and even acne. However, they can be quite unstable because of changes in environmental temperatures and its pH due to exposure. So it is a good idea to use freshly mashed fruit as soon as possible on your skin for maximum benefit.

CHAPTER 2

SKIN STRESSORS

Open pores

THIS IS ONE COMPLAINT that everyone has irrespective of their age, and why not? Even if you have absolutely clean complexion, if the pores are wide open, your skin does not look beautiful. The skin actually starts to look dull because it does not reflect light evenly. When this gets linked with oily skin, comedones (bumps on the skin that give it a rough texture), and acne, you end up hating this condition further. It is important you have your pores nice and closed so that your skin looks flawless and bright.

Why do you get open pores?

Sometimes you are genetically prone to have open pore skin, maybe in combination with oily skin. Then as you age, your skin gets relaxed and the pores open up. Excessively steaming your face during a facial or while body steaming and sauna, or the latest craze of hot yoga, can lead to permanently relaxed pores.

How to deal with it?

The simplest thing you can do is use absolutely chilled water from your fridge and splash it on your face. That acts like an instant toner which tightens up your pores. Also, make sure that every time you go to a salon, ask them to use cool mist after they have done the blackhead extraction and deep cleansing. Ask them to put a cold towel on your face while you are in a steam chamber. Splash cold water on your face after a hot shower. You can use ice cubes wrapped in a bit of muslin on your pores as a cooling pack. You can try a mask with kaolin clay or fuller's earth (multani mitti) to tighten the pores. Apply calamine lotion to calm the skin.

Try mild peels on your own at home. Buy either Kojic Acid 6–20%, Azelaic Acid 10–20%, or Salicylic Acid of around 2%, which are all available over the counter. You can apply them one at a time and leave it overnight and see how your skin takes it. Once your skin gets used to it, you can mix all the three and apply it. Leave it on for a couple of hours and see how your skin reacts. Once it adjusts to the blend, you can leave it overnight. If you have oily skin, use this twice a week, and if your skin is dry, then apply it only once a week. Application of Tretinoin and Retino-A ointments at night over a period of time also helps. Look for pore minimizing creams or serums for wearing under your sunscreen during the day.

At your skin doctor's

You can also go to your doctor's to get mild peels done regularly. Ask for Retin-A peels and medium depth peels. You can do mesotherapy wherein Botox is injected underneath your skin to shrink the pores. You can also opt for collagen remodelling laser treatment which shrinks the pores automatically.

Adult acne

Adult acne is a skin problem that you can face between the ages of 40 to 50. So how do identify that you have adult acne? The first sign of adult acne is that it will appear in your C-Zone. Adult acne presents itself as a tenderness that can start 5 to 7 days before you see an actual pimple on the skin. It gets really red and painful. It may not even become a pustule like teenage acne and just remain there for quite some time, hurting you, and then subside leaving behind a dark mark.

Why do you get adult acne?

Hormonal fluctuation is the culprit. It can be stress related as well. Other signs of hormonal fluctuation include breast tenderness, your menstrual cycle going all haywire, and abnormal hair growth on your chin and other facial areas. Then you know that there's something wrong going on with your hormones. It is usually sporadic.

Alterations in the level of female and male hormones can lead to stimulation of sebaceous glands and hair growth on your face. You might also notice some on your back and chest. These hormones also reduce BMR which increases your tendency to put on weight around your belly. What happens is this—your excess female hormones are converted into male hormones in the peripheral fat which further harms the skin and affects the metabolism of body fat.

The other factor that can trigger adult acne is your thyroid. If you have a family history of thyroid abnormality or going through a stressful situation, then you have higher chances of sprouting pimples. Both these situations can be brought under control; all you need to do is visit your endocrinologist.

Yet another cause could be wrong cosmetic products or make up and any other medication that you may be on. In such a case all you need to do is to stop the application of your beauty product, make up, or medication. Slowly reintroduce them one by one to find out the trigger to the skin irritation. Then go and consult your doctor.

What do you do to deal with it?

You could simply start off with yoga and exercise to make sure that happy hormones are released. It can go a long way in calming you from the inside which then shows on the outside.

At home, start regulating your skincare regime—pick a face wash that matches your needs, regulate your night cream, and check your sunscreen. Start your at-home care with a Salicylic Acid or Benzoyl Peroxide cream. Eat a balanced diet with anti-inflammatory ingredients. You can also take oral anti-inflammatory medication, EFA, and antioxidants.

At your skin doctor's

First get the right medication to regulate your hormones. Then go for gentle peels. You can also opt for certain lasers and light therapy.

Stretch marks

If I had a magic wand that could erase stretch marks, I would be a millionaire by now. But then I don't have the wand, and neither does anybody I know. We all know why we get stretch marks—pregnancy, sudden weight loss—there can be so many reasons for it. But can we really do anything about it? Can we prevent those lines? No. All the creams and all the oils that claim to do so cannot prevent stretch marks if your skin is prone to it. Your genetic make up is responsible for it as well. However, you can ease your skin into it and reduce the severity of the marks.

When you are pregnant and putting on and then losing weight rapidly, lubricate your skin with these special potions:

Calendula: Stimulates growth of new skin cells

Celery oil: Eases congestion, puffiness, and swelling of the skin

Camomile: Has a cooling and soothing effect on the skin

Lavender: Soothing effect on dry and itching skin

Vitamin A: Helps improve the skin's elasticity, texture, and tone

Vitamin E: Increases the moisture content of the epidermis, thereby making the skin softer, smoother, and suppler

But if you have already developed stretch marks, then can you really get rid of them? Sorry, but no, not completely.

Though, with care and certain treatments, you might be able to lighten the appearance and reduce the severity.

Here's what you can do at home

- ✤ Regularly apply the special stretch mark potion
- ✤ Apply Retin-A creams
- ✤ You can use acids and skin lightening creams if you have dark stretch marks

At your skin doctor's

You can opt for peels, laser skin resurfacing, micro-needling and radio frequency. In fact, I have got super results with a combination of all the above.

Hyperpigmentation

Hyperpigmentation is characterized by a darkening of an area of the skin. This is most often caused by overproduction of a pigment called melanin. This overproduction is due to an increase in the number or activity of melanocytes. Though it can occur to a person belonging to any race, those of Asian, Mediterranean, African or Latin origin are more prone to it.

Why do you get hyperpigmentation?

Here are some common forms of hyperpigmentation and their causes:

Tanning: Sun exposure stimulates the production of melanin.

Melasma: Brownish discolouration of the face, more often across the cheek, nose, forehead, and chin areas. It is more common in women and those with a darker complexion. It is associated with hormonal changes like those that occurs during pregnancy (called chloasma), and by the use of oral contraceptives. It is aggravated due to sun exposure and may become permanent with the lack of timely intervention.

Freckles: Small peppery brown spots arising on the face and other sun exposed areas. They darken and increase in number during summer and get lighter during winters.

Lentigenes: Brown to black spots that occur mostly in sun exposed areas; there is no seasonal variation.

Age spots or liver spots: Small, flat, pigmented spots which look similar to freckles. Most often seen on the sun exposed skin after you cross 40; it usually occurs on the face, shoulders, neck, ear, and the back of the hands. Unlike freckles, these generally do not fade with treatment.

Dermatosis Papulosa Nigra or DPN: Small, 1-3mm sized areas of thickened skin that gradually enlarge with time. They are not pre-cancerous.

Mole (Nevus): Growths on the skin that are usually brown or black. They may appear at birth or later in life. A vast majority of moles are benign but some that may be of medical concern are those that develop due to sudden change in the colour, size, or shape; or if they bleed, ooze, itch or become tender or painful; or if they are very large or asymmetric moles.

Skin tag: A small flap of tissue that hangs off the skin by a connecting stalk. They are not dangerous.

Post Inflammatory Hyperpigmentation (PIH): Pigmentation that occurs after any superficial damage to the skin like pimple, superficial burn, cut or abrasion. This leaves a mark that is darker than the rest of the skin.

Pigmentation on other body parts: Pigmentation on the back or upper arms is common in individuals who have darker skin despite the long-term use of body scrubs or loofahs. Pigmentation may occur in those with some hormonal disorders like Addison's disease, caused by adrenal insufficiency; Cushing's disease, those with insulin resistance; Acanthosis Nigricans, hyperpigmentation of intertriginous areas and body folds; Grave's disease, thyroid disorder. In addition, patients of certain liver or kidney diseases or certain kinds of vitamin deficiencies or some underlying malignancy may also develop hyperpigmentation on various body parts. Certain fungal infections may also cause the skin to look patchy or dry. Chronic friction may also cause pigmentation of certain body parts like the chin or neck due to regular threading, or elbows or knees due to posture.

The pigment cycle

Skin cells that make melanin are in the lowermost layer of the epidermis. With age, melanocyte distribution becomes less controlled, causing dark spots to form instead of clear, even skin.

Name of the pigmentary condition	Melasma	Sunspots/ Age spots/ Liver Spots	Post-inflammatory hyper-pigmentation (PIH)	Freckles
Colour	Light to medium brown	Light to dark brown	Brown to black	Light to dark brown or black
Place of occurrence	On the cheeks, sides of the face, upper part of the nose, forehead, and above the lip	On the face, chest, and hands, not much in darker individuals	Anywhere	On the face, chest and arms
What it looks like	Patches that are inconsistent in shape and size	Small, flat, dark spots	Flat spots or raised	Concentrated small spots, seasonal variation
Cause	A surge in hormones, usually from pregnancy or birth control coupled with sun exposure, may run in the family	The sun	Any skin injury, trauma, friction, pressure, lasers, inflammatory acne etc.	The sun, genetic

Name of the pigmentary condition	Melasma	Sunspots/ Age spots/ Liver Spots	Post-inflammatory hyper-pigmentation (PIH)	Freckles
How to treat it?	Hydroquinone and Retin-A; Azelic, Salicylic, Lactic or Glycolic Acid peels, Q-switched Nd Yag laser; or hard to treat, may come back with a vengeance	Retinol + IPL fractional laser	Light Salicylic Acid chemical peels; lasers. avoid causing factors	Q switched Nd Yag laser at 532 nm

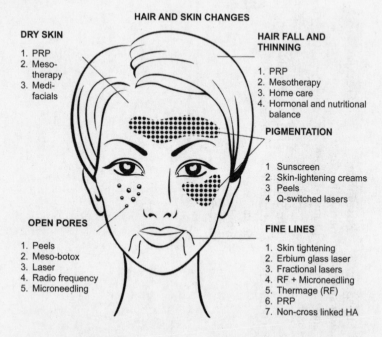

HAIR AND SKIN CHANGES

DRY SKIN

1. PRP
2. Meso-
   therapy
3. Medi-
   facials

HAIR FALL AND THINNING

1. PRP
2. Mesotherapy
3. Home care
4. Hormonal and nutritional balance

PIGMENTATION

1 Sunscreen
2 Skin-lightening creams
3 Peels
4 Q-switched lasers

OPEN PORES

1. Peels
2. Meso-botox
3. Laser
4. Radio frequency
5. Microneedling

FINE LINES

1. Skin tightening
2. Erbium glass laser
3. Fractional lasers
4. RF + Microneedling
5. Thermage (RF)
6. PRP
7. Non-cross linked HA

Step 01

Melanin production is triggered.

Sun exposure, inflammation, or a hormonal surge, trigger a signal to the hormones that control melanin production. Once this signal is sent, the enzyme tyrosinase tells the body to start the process of creating more melanin.

Step 02

The melanocyte cells start producing a new pigment.

This newly created pigment is then packaged into little bundles called melanosomes.

Step 03

Pigment is distributed.

Next, the melanosomes disperse the pigment through the dermis up to the epidermis through their dendrites. If the pigment doesn't make its way up toward the surface and stay in the dermis, they will be harder to erase.

The cause of dark spots

The Sun: UV rays produce excess melanin, which is deposited in the skin.

Inflammation: Trauma to the skin is one of the main causes for hyperpigmentation, and also responsible for sharp, blunt or normal irritation and inflammation.

Acne: The more severe the blemish the more inflammed the skin is, and the more likely it is to pigment. Inflamed areas naturally produce more melanin.

Hormones: Pregnancy, birth control, and menopause can cause a spike in melanin production.

Lasers and peels: Laser and strong chemical peels cause inflammation, and the body may respond with brown patches or stripes.

Medication: Some antibiotics (sulphonamides and tetracyclines) and medications to treat Parkinson's disease, cancer, diabetes, and heart disease, can lead to dark patches as an allergic reaction or because of increased sun sensitivity.

Regardless of what caused your skin to become uneven in tone, the slightest bit of sun exposure (mere minutes in the sun can be enough for some) can trigger the skin to kick melanin production into overdrive. That's why wearing sunscreen daily is stressed in almost all the sections.

> 'Akshara and I have always believed in home-care from natural ingredients. And now that both Akshara and I are shooting, using make up, and are constantly exposed to the sun, skincare routine—cleansing and protection against the sun—is a must. Sun protection, I feel, is of utmost importance not only to look beautiful but also for protection against skin ailments.'
>
> Sarika, Actress

Surface pigmentation vs. deep pigmentation

When pigmentation is on the top most layer of your skin, the discolouration is more of a light brown colour and is more diffused. It also responds better to treatment. Pigmentation deep within skin takes on more of a dark brown or grey shade and is solid and hence harder to treat.

Chemical peels

These are a series of light 'chemical' peels that use Salicylic Acid, Lactic Acid, Glycolic Acid, resorcinol, TCA, Jessner's solution etc. They can improve skin texture and colour.

Laser resurfacing treatments and intense pulsed light (IPL)

Laser treatments—in which a beam of fractionated energy is delivered to skin to incite a wound-healing response—can work wonders to correct hyperpigmentation or more specifically sunspots and acne scars. When using lasers to treat hyperpigmentation, it is important that a low-energy, non-ablative fractional laser is used. Otherwise, new or more pigmentation can develop. Nd: YAG lasers can also be used to treat spots.

Enzymes

Enzymes are tiny little proteins that accelerate chemical reactions in skin cells and on the surface of the skin, they are responsible for softening it. They also dissolve and digest old, dry skin cells so that you can wash them away easily to reveal healthy, glowing skin.

Enzymes tend to be gentler than acids in chemically loosening the cells of your outer most layer. Enzymes are less acidic and have a pH value closer to the skin's natural state. Every fruit has an enzyme and all of them can help, so you can simply use the pulp to massage or apply it as a pack and let it stay on for 15 minutes.

The upside

Since many enzymes are derived from fruits, they also up the ante by being antioxidants and having the ability to scavenge free radicals. They also help jump-start cell turnover and boost the metabolism of cells to help keep skin acting young.

The downside

Enzymes can break down very quickly—many of us could be allergic to them. I am allergic to aloe vera. And if you are looking for a specific benefit, you may not really achieve it as the actives may not be potent enough.

Papin (Papaya): Very powerful exfoliator and anti-inflammatory.

Protease (Pumpkin): In addition to its exfoliating ability, it also has anti-ageing superstar vitamin A.

Bromelain (Pineapple): anti-inflammatory

Malic Acid (Green Apples): Although it's found in several fruits, malic acid is most abundant in green apples.

Actinidin (Kiwi Fruit): A vitamin-C powerhouse that also has the ability to brighten the skin. Kiwi fruit is perhaps the most suitable enzyme for sensitive skin.

For more information on skin, you can visit my webpage http://www.drrashmishetty.com/pages/skin.html

CHAPTER 3

HORMONES AND SKIN

Not just your mood swings, bloating, and PMS; hormones play with your skin and hair too

ONCE YOU CROSS THE age of 30, you will notice many changes in your body—especially your skin and hair. This is impacted by the changing state of the hormones in your body. Having a full understanding of how hormones—and the lack of them—affect your skin is important if you want to maintain great skin and hair.

Hormones are chemical messengers that are produced in organs such as the ovaries, adrenal glands, and thyroid glands. Sex steroid hormones, thyroid and growth hormones are involved in many different functions such as growth, immune, reproductive and metabolic functions, and even hunger and stress. Many factors are involved in intrinsic skin ageing like genetic mutations, increased inflammatory signals, decreased lipid production, and decreased hormone levels.

One of the most important factors involved in the initiation of your ageing process is the endocrine system.

The endocrine system produces and regulates hormones. It is important for you to have a healthy endocrine system because for women its decline, sometimes drastically, with age, can impact you severely. This is simply because it directly impacts the state of hormones in your body.

As a result, you might start noticing dryness, fine lines and pale skin, and thinning of hair. Now, let us closely monitor the hormonal changes since we have learnt how important they are for healthy skin, especially for women. Here are some hormones that you need know about to understand how they affect your skin and hair as you grow older.

Oestrogen

When it comes to popular hormones, oestrogen takes the prize. It is often called the hormone of beauty—it is responsible for the shape of your body and the state of your hair and skin. With progesterone, oestrogen controls the functions of your reproductive organs.

It is primarily made in the ovaries and also in different tissues outside of the ovaries. Oestrogen actually encompasses a group of chemically similar hormones, so it is not a single substance. Oestrogens include estradiol, the most abundant form in adult females; estriol, the primary oestrogen during pregnancy; and estrone, which is produced during menopause.

Oestrogens affect skin thickness, wrinkle formation, and skin moisture. Oestrogens can increase glycosaminoglycans (GAGs) such as Hyaluronic Acid. They can also increase collagen production in the skin, where they maintain epidermal thickness and allow the skin to remain plump, hydrated, and wrinkle-free.

During periods of elevated hormonal activity, such as pregnancy or while on oral contraceptives, skin pigmentation is exacerbated in certain sun-exposed areas such as the forehead, nose, and cheeks. This phenomenon, known as melasma, is strictly hormone-related and is a clear example of hormonal effects on skin pigmentation.

Your skin is not the only external feature that benefits from oestrogens. Besides resulting in plump, healthy skin, oestrogens can also make hair grow long and healthy. So during pregnancy, you will experience hair growth which is thick and lustrous because the excess oestrogen in your body improves the stable phase of your hair or Anagen. However postpartum and during menopause, the drop in estrogenic levels cause thinning and falling hair, sometimes resulting in clinically significant hair loss, or the Telogen Effluvium.

In essence, oestrogens help our skin and hair remain youthful. Of course, during puberty, menstruation, and menopause, progesterone plays a key role. However, research is still going on in this field. Future research will hopefully shed some light on the interactions between oestrogens and progesterone and help us better understand these changes in our skin and hair.

Progesterone

Progesterone is a hormone that stimulates and regulates various functions in our body. It plays a major role in maintaining healthy pregnancy in women. It regulates the monthly menstrual cycle and prepares your body for conception. This hormone is produced in the ovaries, placenta (the organ that helps transfer nourishment from a pregnant mother to the baby), and the adrenals. High progesterone levels can cause PMS in women; you will notice tenderness in your breasts, bloating, and even mood swings. It also impacts skin by tightening the connective tissues and it is also responsible for remodelling the collagen structure.

Testosterone

Testosterone is the chief male sex hormone that defines all the masculine characteristics in a man. Coarser hair, thicker and oilier skin, and generally a later onset of signs of skin ageing are all due to testosterone. Female pattern alopecia or baldness, is attributed to increased androgen levels and is the most common cause of hair loss in women. Androgens are the hormones that lead to hair fall in genetically predisposed individuals.

With age, the oestrogen-androgen ratio becomes unbalanced, and changes are seen following menopause. Since androgens, and in particular testosterone, are involved in sebum production, females may experience increased oiliness or even adult acne when hormones become unbalanced during menstruation or menopause. Androgens affect both males and females and they can experience the effects of altered androgen levels.

Thyroid Hormones

The thyroid is a small butterfly-shaped gland situated just in front of the voice box. The thyroid gland makes two thyroid hormones which affect metabolism, brain development, breathing, body temperature, muscle strength, bone health, skin dryness, menstrual cycles, weight, and cholesterol levels. Again, balance is key when it comes to these hormones. Too much of it and the skin can become warm, sweaty, and flushed. Too little of it can make the skin dry, coarse, thick and even reduce the sweating. Thyroid dysfunction can also lead to the thinning of hair and eventual hair loss.

DHEA (Dehydroepiandrosterone)

DHEA (dehydroepiandrosterone) is called the 'mother hormone' because it acts as a precursor to other hormones in the body such as oestrogen, progesterone, cortisone, androgen, and testosterone, to name a few. It is an important endogenous steroid hormone. It is naturally produced by the adrenal glands, the gonads, and the brain. Levels of DHEA naturally drop once you cross 30.

What happens when your hormones go haywire?

- ❖ The variations in your hormones can lead to discolouration of skin. The melanocytes, which are the basis of skin's pigment, get affected with changes in pituitary hormones and thyroid hormones.
- ❖ Excessive male hormones in your body can affect the sebaceous glands and lead to adult acne.
- ❖ Also when DHEA and androsterones turn into testosterones, they become DHT or Dihydrotestosterones. DHT is responsible for increasing male pattern baldness in women. It constricts the roots and hurts the hair follicles leading to thin strands.

- ❖ Unopposed increase in male hormones also leads to hair growth on the chin and the upper lip region.
- ❖ As oestrogen drops, your body starts to lose its capacity to absorb calcium.
- ❖ When hormones start to retire their functions, various bodily functions like sexual desire, state of skin and hair, bone density, and physical and intellectual capabilities start to degrade.
- ❖ The first sign that there is some hormonal change taking place in your body is that your sleep pattern gets disturbed, the release of melatonin—sleep hormones—get affected, and the rest follows. This also leads to decrease in the multiplication of epidermal cells, decrease in oil glands leading to dry skin, and often large pores. As the bone density starts to decrease, the structure of your face alters.

Menopause

Menopause, as the name suggests, is the suspension of woman hormones for good. These days women attain menopause by the time they are 45, if not earlier. This is all thanks to the lifestyle, stress, food habits, pollution, and hormones in our daily lives.

What happens during menopause to your skin and hair?

The onslaught of menopause leads to low oestrogen levels, causing:

- ❖ Excessive drying of skin hydration and mucous membrane. So you get flaky, dry, sensitive and itchy skin, dry lips and vagina, dry nails with longitudinal ridges.

- ✤ Decreased collagen synthesis and increased destruction of its structure, leading to accelerated skin ageing.
- ✤ Decreased cell turnover and sloughing making the skin look dull and darker.
- ✤ Alteration in thermoregulation—hot flushes, redness on your face, or exacerbation of conditions like acne or rosacea.
- ✤ Melasma—pigmentation on your cheeks, forehead, nose, and upper lip.
- ✤ Unopposed action of male hormones—excessive hair on the chin, hair thinning, or hairfall.
- ✤ Fat resorption from the face—sagging of the soft tissue.
- ✤ Decreased calcium absorption, bone resorption, causes structural collapse of the face.

How to deal with this?

If you have been taking good care of your skin, by the time you hit 35, your skin will not go through major lows. You can up your moisturizer though and buy creams with special anti-ageing actives. You have to take special care of your skin with gentle treatment products. Since the body metabolism slows down, some stretching exercises to deal with spot weight gain can also help. You also need to workout to keep your joints and bones healthy. You can seek professional help to reduce fine lines, and moisturize your skin.

You could just be suffering from iron deficiency. Even if you are not anaemic and your haemoglobin is within normal limits, the elemental iron could be low. Check your serum ferritin and B12; Ferritin should be between 80 and 100. The cause for dark circles and hair fall could just be this and it is treatable.

Hair woes

Thinning hair and hair fall is another problem that crops up as you hit menopause. Many of my patients come to me not for skin but hair woes. As you grow older, your hair starts to get dry and scanty. The texture gets fine and becomes more susceptible to breakage and of course it goes grey. None of that is complementary to our looks.

You can definitely start colouring your hair. Look for an ammonia-free colour which is much more gentle on the strands. Go easy on the blow dry. Avoid heavy-duty irons and dryers at the salon. Oiling your hair, especially a good scalp massage, is a good thing to being with if you have not been doing so. Do not forget take your daily supplements.

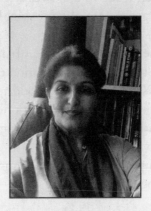

DR RANJANA DHANU, GYNAECOLOGIST

Dr Dhanu was one of the first doctors who supported me when I was still finding my way in the industry. She also happens to be my gynaecologist who took care of me during my pregnancy. Thank you for being a part of my journey and for all the yummy food.

Dr Dhanu's gyan

IF YOU ARE 35 and your skin, mood, and body has already started to bother you much more than it did before, welcome to the 'climacteric' phase meaning pre-menopause,which leads to a slowdown of your ovaries. You must take special care of your skin, body, and bones now.

So what is menopause? It is the permanent cessation of ovarian activity along with cessation of menstruation. You confirm this with a simple blood test—check your levels of follicle stimulating hormone (FSH) which should be 20 and above. The average age of menopause is between 42 to 53 years.

The most important thing that turns your world around is oestrogen sinking.

Early effects of reduced oestrogen

- Mood swings, depression due to increase in encephalins—the sad hormones and endorphins—that lower the happy hormones.
- Sex drive, i.e. libido decreases.
- Thermoregulatory system goes haywire causing hot flushes.
- Maldistribution of the fat. Your breast flattens, belly girth increases, and facial fat descends.
- Your basal metabolic rate (BMR) goes down. You realize that while your food intake hasn't changed, the fat retained is lot more.
- Vaginal dryness as mucus membrane thins too. This means painful intercourse and repeated UTIs, also called UroGenital Syndrome.

❖ Stress incontinence wherein when you cough or lift weight, a little bit of your urine escapes.

As you start to notice the changes, try supplements that can help you. The popular ones are vitamin D3, calcium, primrose oil, and multivitamins that help you have an easy menopause.

The long-term effects

❖ Alzheimer's
❖ Cardiovascular changes
❖ Bone density changes leading to osteoporosis

The National Osteoporosis Foundation recommends you take:

❖ 500mg of calcium once a day if you are 35 and above.
❖ At menopause and thereafter, 1000mg of calcium in a day.
❖ When you are 65 and above then 1500mg of calcium in a day along with exercise.

Dr Dhanu says that the WHO recommendation is that a doctor can give HRT only if the patient is symptomatic after all the investigations have been done and all the protocols have been met with.

Do phytoestrogens work?

No they don't. Phytoestrogens are plant derivatives that many claim, if taken in form of supplements, act like oestrogens, but don't fall for it. They are just placebos.

CHAPTER 4

SKINCARE EMERGENCIES

WHEN I OPTED FOR aesthetic skincare as my speciality in medicine, I never thought I'd have a 'real emergency' to deal with. Remember times when your skin breaks out into a huge red zit just a day before your most important function? It's panic, panic, panic. It's a skin emergency! Some skin emergencies that most of us have to deal with at some point or the other are:

Super sensitive skin

This happens when your skin gets extremely dehydrated and dry—chapped, burning, and red. All you have to do is a quick cold water face wash. Use a creamy variant. Then on slightly damp face apply a cold cream—a really thick layer of rich and creamy cold cream. Make sure it has no active ingredients in it, which means it should not be a skin lightening or an anti-ageing cream. When you apply the cream, it might cause slight irritation. But don't worry, keep it on. It will calm your skin down.

If the condition is really bad, use desonide lotion, which is a very mild steroid, safe even for baby's nappy rash. Mix that with a calamine lotion that comes pre-mixed with a moisturizer. It will ensure that your face does not dry up. Apply that and it will calm your skin. You can use this same solution if your skin goes red.

Itchy skin

It could be a reaction to a new cosmetic that you have applied, or an old, expired cosmetic, an infected brush, a moist make up sponge which tends to gather bacteria, something in your food, the dust around you, or a mite bite. First, rule out the reason which could have given you the condition. Take an antihistamine like Allegra or Cetirizine, which calms your skin from the inside. Go take a good head shower so that your scalp is clean. Then wash your face with a soothing face wash so that your face feels clean. After this, apply a mixture of desonide and calamine lotion. That will take care of itchiness for the moment; if the condition does not improve, then rush to your doctor immediately for medical help. If you have itching in your tongue or throat, or if you notice puffiness around your eyes, lips, or have difficulty breathing, leave everything else and rush to your nearest doctor.

Sudden breakage of zits

Firstly calm down, because the more you stress, the more they are likely to occur. Wash you face with cold water, and keep a couple of ointments handy like Bactroban and Safrodex (which is a mix of antibiotic and steroid).

Dot it on top of the zit and it will most likely calm down. However, if it looks little red and flushed, like it will not go down in a day, use Benzoyl Peroxide gel or cream. But make sure you don't apply too much of it as that can make the skin red around the acne. Just dot it on the acne.

If the zit is too big, and there's pus in it, then buy a sterile needle from a chemist and very lightly poke it right on top, and let the pus ooze out. Don't push too hard, and make sure you don't use your nails to scratch it out. If you squeeze it, you might drive the pus right into the zit and may end up with an abscess. Apply ice to calm it down.

A tan that burns

After long sun exposure, you must take special care. So first wash your skin with cold water, and then apply plenty of moisturizer and calamine lotion. It is important to calm the skin first. Then after a couple of days, use special treatment creams that lighten the skin like glycolic acid, kojic acid, apply it at night so that the tan slowly comes off. You can have a slightly long shower, and then use a towel against that natural grain of your skin to slough off dead skin. You will see the dead skin literally come off, and with that the tan comes off to pretty much a large extent. Do not use a scrub immediately after sunburn because it will make your skin further flushed and reactive.

Products to keep

1. Calamine lotion with moisturizer
2. T-bact, Sofradex ointment
3. Desonide ointment—a mild skin healing steroid.
4. Rich creamy moisturizer
5. Ice cubes—the wonder tool to deal with all skin issues like redness, burning, and even acne
6. Kojic acid or Glycolic acid cream to take off pigmentation
7. Anti-histamine like Allegra or Cetrizine
8. Sandalwood paste
9. Cold milk

Help at home

My mother's favourite recipe to all skin woes is sandalwood paste. Get a piece of sandalwood, which most of us South Indians have at home. Rub it on a rough wet stone and use tender coconut water as the medium. Mix that with milk or milk cream and turmeric. Apply on your face or body. It will soothe, calm, heal, and lighten the skin. It is a one shot cure-all for your skin.

CHAPTER 5

WHILE YOU ARE SLEEPING

YOU MUST GET YOUR 6–8 hours beauty sleep every night. Trust me, beauty sleep—real, deep slumber—is nature's best defence against skin ageing. I can't stress enough on the importance of getting the right amount of sleep. Research has shown that there is a direct correlation between the number of hours you sleep and how your skin looks and feels.

As your body rests, the skin repairs itself. When you slip into the second phase of your sleep at night—what we call the delta phase—your hormone levels are at their peak, and that's when cell repair takes place.

So what happens really is that any damage to the collagen and elastin under your skin that might have taken place due to say free radicals can be repaired as you sleep. Free radicals, as I have said earlier, is one of the biggest culprits in premature ageing.

Want glowing skin? Then hit the bed every night at around the same time, and sleep. Give your skin cells time to rest, repair, and restore. If it's only 5 hours you can manage every night, then it's better to sleep early and wake up early than to sleep late and wake up later

Deep sleep = Radiant complexion

Lack of sleep constricts the blood vessels on your face. It looks dull, and lacklustre. Sleep actually helps in collagen production. And you need loads of that for skin that's supple and elastic.

Do you feel tautness in your skin when you wake up? That happens when your skin loses hydration at night when you sleep. All that repair work underneath tends to pull out water from the top layer that is if your air conditioner spares some.

To do: Drink at least a glass of water before going to bed and apply a hydrating moisturizer to ensure that your skin does not lose hydration from the outside.

Deep sleep + vitamin enriched night cream = Supple, line-free skin

You can actually help your skin in its repairing efforts by adding some extra dose of vitamins and essential skin actives. When you wake up your skin will thank you for it. I am sure you will also feel very nice about it too.

Deep sleep + anti-wrinkle under eye cream = smooth toned, clear sparkling eyes

Nothing like a good night's sleep to fight puffy eyes and dark circles. I am sure you have noticed that after a good night's sleep your eyes look bright, and the under eye area looks smooth and toned. We Indian girls tend to suffer from uneven skin tone, especially under the eyes. This is something you can take care of as you sleep. A little care goes a long way.

To do: Buy a lightening under eye cream—look for ingredients like liquorice and vitamin E. Don't rub, but dab the cream in circular motion around the area. Go to sleep and wake up with prettier eyes. Go low on salt after sunset. You can also put two pillows to prop yourself. Sleep on your back and not on your sides or stomach.

Your pre-sleep prepping routine

- Remove make up, and cleanse your face with a cleanser. Use soft cotton pressed pads to wipe away the dirt.
- Use a face wash to wash off the residue. Exfoliate if you feel the need.
- Go for deep cleansing shower/bath with exfoliating body wash.
- Use a muslin cloth/ towel to dab your face and body. It retains water in the skin without leaving it wet.
- Put on your under eye cream, dab and leave it to soak into the skin.
- Apply an AHA-based hand and body lotion. Slather it on nicely. Massage gently till the lotion soaks in. Apply your foot cream as well.
- Massage a rich night cream all over your face, neck, and décolletage in upward and circular motion.
- Drink a glass of warm water before going to bed.

The Sleep Pattern

First three hours: You get the deepest sleep of the night. Your body produces the most human growth hormones, which are crucial to skin and hair repair.

Middle two hours: Deep sleep shortens and rapid eye movement (REM) sleep begins. Melatonin, a hormone that's also a skin-protecting antioxidant, increases.

Last three hours: This is when you get the most REM sleep. Your skin's temperature reaches its lowest point and your muscles relax, giving your skin its deepest recovery.

CHAPTER 6

SKIN AND WEATHER

I HAVE OFTEN HAD patients come to me with a pre-conceived notion of what their skin state is in. Sometimes it really takes lots of patience and talking before I can make them see sense. You need to understand that the state of your skin is never constant, especially if you are a woman who goes out to work and spends time in different environmental conditions.

The external conditions—pollutants, dirt, grime, and changing weather—play a major role in how your skin feels or behaves. You might be born with a certain type of skin, but over the course of time, weather changes can aggravate a skin condition or change its texture. I am sure you must have noticed that if your skin is prone to oiliness, summer time can be a pain because suddenly the greasy skin factor increases tenfold. Similarly, if in normal conditions your skin is dry, it looks dull, flaky, and dehydrated in winter.

You need to examine your current skincare regimen and adjust it to meet your skin's ever changing needs based on shifts in climate and sun levels. It's especially critical to establish (and diligently follow) a routine that meets your skin's specific needs during specific climatic conditions.

Also just to highlight that with many of us jet-setting now across the globe, say in the span of one week, your skin faces different conditions. For instance, you may start off from a summer country and land in winter into another. While you do your travel packing, make sure your skincare products are packed accordingly. Your skincare routine must remain the same but according to the changing climate conditions, you must use specific products.

Do not go by what you think is your skin type to choose products round the year. Be tuned in to the changes in the weather and how your skin reacts to it. Once you start recording the changes, you will naturally be in sync and treat your skin accordingly. Change your face washes, cleansers, moisturizer, and sun protection products to match your skin condition at a particular moment. You will be surprised that all it really takes is to just do these adjustments in your daily regime to keep your skin perfect and glowing round the year without any special skincare treatments.

Summer

Soaring temperatures and high humidity leave, your skin sticky, oily, and dull with wide open pores. In summer, cleaning your skin thoroughly should become your main focus. Dirt and grime sticking to skin can make it look unhealthy and lifeless, and you will look tired. A clean skin without blocked pores and acne makes you look fresh and beautiful. Remember, staying indoors does not necessarily protect you from UV rays.

Look and feel of summer skin

- ❖ Oily, sticky, and dark
- ❖ Wide open pores
- ❖ Acne prone
- ❖ Frizzed out hair and sticky scalp
- ❖ Excessive sweating
- ❖ For men: Dark, oily, and excessively sweaty face and scalp

Summer special care

Face wash, your key ritual: In summer, getting a squeaky clean face should be your main beauty ritual. Take off your make up first with a good make up remover. Choosing the right face wash is THE most important thing in summer. Choose a face wash that lathers, feels fresh, minty, and light. Look for fruit acids, mint and tea-tree in your face wash. If you are acne prone, then salicylic acid and benzoyl peroxide are the actives to look out for.

If you are out the whole day and do not have time to wash your face, you could either use a face wipe or spray a face mist liberally on your face and wipe it with a clean tissue. Don't forget to reapply sunscreen. By doing this you can avoid removing your eye and lip make up.

Use a toner if you like: Even though using a toner is not my favourite must dos, you can always give it a try. If you can lay your hands on a toner that does not dry your skin but makes you feel clean, then use it. Put some on a soft cotton pad and wipe your face with it. Warmer weather can mean more 'shine' (when the skin is oily) than 'glow' (which comes from healthy skin) for oily or combination complexions. If you miss the fresh feeling you got with your toner, then I suggest you pick up mists. Rosewater works wonders too. You can keep some in the fridge to make a cool skin-pick-me-up or to soothe irritated skin.

Exfoliating the right way: In summers, I recommend you use a scrub only once a week. When you are using any form of exfoliator, you are attempting to remove the top dead layer of the skin, which is a not such a good idea. This top dead layer is actually your protecting layer which will help you against sun damage.

Excessive scrubbing can make the skin more sensitive, red, and vulnerable. And even the once-a-week scrub should be done gently and at night. Immediately put on a soothing agent. Make sure the size of the granules are very small and skin friendly. In fact, a few popular scrubs, which at times my patients tell me are their favourite, is something I won't even recommend as a foot scrub!

I scream sunscreen: These days, with all the BB and CC creams coming up, there are day creams with multiple ingredients and benefits. But, in summer, the one and only important goal is to protect yourself against sunlight and keep your skin hydrated and yet not oily. Sunscreen is your best friend now. Even day creams with SPF 20 is a good option.

When I speak about sunscreen in summer, the two complaints I hear are that it makes you look dark and sticky and at times it leads to acne. And these days there are enough sunscreens that are well formulated and non-oily or do not leave a white residue after application. The darkness that you see is because of your skin getting greasy. If you wash your face every four hours, you can still look bright and beautiful with the sunscreen on. Make sure you re-apply your sunscreen after each wash.

Supplement with serums: In summer, most of your skin concerns like pigmentation, acne, and skin tightening, can be addressed with the active ingredients in a serum form or gel form. This is because they have the actives in water or silicon base which do not add to the oiliness. You could either apply them in the evening or underneath your sunscreen during the day.

After-sun care: A day out at the beach under the hot sun is fun, but it can also harm your skin greatly. As soon as you get back, wash your face with chilled water, use a soothing lotion, and do not use harsh treatment creams that night. Peeling agents and scrubs are an absolute no-no! What looks red today can turn black tomorrow. You can also apply a cooling after-sun gel that has ingredients like cucumber, aloe vera, or green tea. This will soothe the redness. You can also try applying grated and chilled cucumber or raw potato slices to calm and soothe the burns.

Skincare for night time: If you are in a humid city like Mumbai, and not using an AC, then simply wash your face with chilled water before going to bed. If you must, then use a calamine lotion. But if you are sleeping with the AC on, and are not in a very humid place, I would recommend you use skin milk or a lotion that calms your skin and adds the much-needed hydration.

Help your hair: Wash your hair every single day to get squeaky clean scalp and hair. Be careful to use the right shampoo and conditioner.

OILY HAIR

Oily hair signifies an oily scalp and is due to excess oil secretion from your scalp which usually leads to dermatitis /dandruff. Dandruff doesn't presents itself like that show in the TV ad, plenty white flakes on your black shirt. It could just be your hair getting excessively oily soon after a bath, or then the next day. In such a case, an anti-dandruff shampoo is your best bet.

- Make sure you use the anti-dandruff shampoo every day for 15 days at least so that you can stop the build-up of free fatty acids on the scalp.
- Then wash it every alternate day. You must remember that dandruff is a long-term issue.
- If you have long hair, use your favourite shampoo for the rest of your hair and apply the anti-dandruff shampoo only on the scalp.
- If you need two rinses, then first use the cosmetic shampoo and then the anti-dandruff one.
- You need to lather it up and let it stay on the scalp for 3 minutes.

- You can condition your hair after following all these steps.

Dry/brittle/damaged hair

- Shampoo should be mild.
- Label should mention hydrating oils like Moroccan /argen/coconut etc.
- Look for protein content.
- A conditioner or a hair cream or mask is a must.
- Take a quick shower with lukewarm water.
- Do not rinse your hair more than once however good your shampoo is.
- Rinse a maximum of two times if you have soaked your hair with oil.

Factors affecting hair follicle

- Normal ageing process
- Oxidative stress
- Lack of proteins
- Inflammation
- UV radiation
- Smoking
- General nutrition and health
- Pollution

Factors affecting the hair shaft

- Excessive combing, or using the wrong brush (as in bristles that are too close and not well aligned) with rough bristles.
- Excessive heat—while blow drying or ironing hair.
- UV rays, pollution in the air, or wind.
- Chemical treatments.

✤ Using wrong hair accessories and bath products.

Do not forget the age-old ritual of oiling. Often, my male patients come to me and tell me that they wash hair every day, but shampoo it every alternate day. Till date, I have not understood this funda. Shampoos are not harmful. They are meant to clean your scalp as a face wash is meant to clean your face. As you wash your face every day with a face wash, so you can shampoo your hair every day to cleanse unnecessary secretions and grime. There are many good variants of shampoos available in the market today to meet your specific hair needs.

Have you noticed how your hair colour fades off in summer or after a beach holiday? Much is spoken about sunscreen for skin, but you would be surprised how much damage the UV rays can do to your hair. There are specific hair care gels and shampoos available for sun protection. Try to use one of those sunscreen hair sprays post shampoo. The best way to protect your hair from harsh UV rays is to wear a hat or a scarf.

Body care: Take a couple of showers during the day using a refreshing body wash and a good deodorant mist to keep the body and mind calm. Use the sunscreen on your body, as it can burn and tan too.

Excessive sweating: If you sweat a lot in restricted body parts, Botox is hugely beneficial.

Botox injections temporarily block the chemical signals from the nerves that stimulate the sweat glands. When the sweat glands don't receive chemical signals, the production of excessive sweat stops in the treated areas and continues to be produced elsewhere. Results last for around 6 months and you do not experience any compensatory sweating anywhere else in the body.

Its procedure is very simple and doctors use tiny injections in the area where you sweat most—palms, soles, underarms etc.

You could use special application products that have anti-perspirant actives like aluminum chloride or aluminum sesquichlorohydrate, or aluminum zirconium trichlorohydrex.

Magic mist: Mist can magically transform your skin. It calms, tones, freshens, and hydrates your skin without making it oily or leaving any heavy residue. You can us it any way you like, under or over make up/sunscreen or as it is. It is the most versatile product out there.

The magic of ice and chilled water

In summer, use only cold water to wash your face. Refrigerate some water and use it as a face wash. Cold water instantly calms your skin and reduces the sun damage, decreases any sort of irritation and shrinks the pores. Also a good idea is to use chilled water before make up and before you set out for the day. This acts as a toner as well. During summers, it is a good idea to store your skincare products, especially your skin soothing agents, in the fridge.

Supplements to take in summer (please consult your doctor/physician before taking them)

➢ Get your daily dose of antioxidants. Take new age antioxidants like Coenzyme Q10, Superoxide Dismutase.

➢ Take vitamins A, C, and E which also act as antioxidants. All of these cut oxidative damage in your body and act as internal sunscreens.

➢ Go high on things that have anti-inflammatory agents like Omega-3 oils. Take one or two capsules of Omega-3, cod liver oil, or primrose oil in a day depending on your dietary intake of oils and your skin/hair condition.

➢ Fruits and vegetables of different colours.

➢ Increase your fluid intake—include buttermilk, coconut water, vegetable juice, clear soups along with water in your daily diet.

Will oil supplements make you fat?

When I ask my patients to take any of the supplements, especially the ones with Omega-3, they worry about whether they will put on weight. Absolutely not!

Summer kitchen goodies

❖ Cucumber eye pack.

❖ Rosewater and sandalwood pack for a toned face.

❖ Milk and yogurt for soothing sunburn and tanned skin.

❖ A tall glass of watermelon and mint juice to cool down your insides.

- Ice is your best friend for summer. Freeze rosewater or tender coconut water into ice cubes. Apply on the face when skin is red/hot—like when you come back from a sunny day, after cooking/workouts, or even when skin pores are open—may be first thing in the day or before applying make up. All you have to do is rub it on the face till the cube melts.
- Stock calamine lotion in the fridge.

At your skin doctor's

TO-DO

- Calming refreshing facial like oxygen facial.
- MesoBotox for open pores.
- Botox for hyperhidrosis (excessive sweating).
- Hair removal lasers (if not actively tanning).
- Radio frequency for skin tightening.

TO AVOID

- Harsh procedures that tamper the top layer of the skin
- Peels
- Microdermabrasion
- Skin lightening laser
- Skin resurfacing laser

Monsoon

Who doesn't love the rains? After the scorching sun and all that dust, it is a relief to feel those drops on your face pouring from the sky. I do enjoy a cup of steaming coffee as the rain lashes around, cooling and cleaning everything. There is such a sense of freshness. But I cannot say the same for the skin. Monsoon brings with it a series of skin woes for many—open pores, dull skin, and infection along body folds. In simpler words, it is summer skin + increased humidity. A bit of moisture is good, but a lot is not.

Look and feel of monsoon

Skin feels hot and humid since the pores are still open from the summer months and can get further aggravated. Acne and skin infection along the body folds can also occur. Sweating can be even more irritating in the humid weather.

Hair swells and so it is more vulnerable to damage i.e. breakage, so is advisable to not go for too many salon treatments. Even a simple blow dry can cause more damage.

Monsoon special care

- Refreshing face wash: Do it four times and with cold water
- Toner: Optional
- Scrub: Once a week
- Day cream: Use only a sunscreen
- Apply skin actives in the form of serums and gels
- Post summer care: Tan removing creams and skin soothing ones
- Night care: Skin lightening actives, AHA and BHA (Acids at 6–20 % are available OTC)
- Just hydrant minus the cream; Magic mist

    ❖ Hair and scalp: Sun protection for hair
    ❖ Body: Couple of showers a day

Pick powders: For this season you must look for the powder form of most things like compact, deodorants etc. There are some collagen boosters in powder form too, which I would suggest you to pick up for keeping your skin in good shape.

Dry up ASAP: If you happen to get wet, wash your face and feet as soon as you can. Keep them dry. A good idea is to carry some wet wipes and then reapply your skincare product or make up.

Stay with sunscreen: If you are planning to cool off on the sunscreen regimen thinking that the clouds will protect you, you are greatly mistaken. The cloudy skies do not guard you from the sun. You can look for a light textured version of suncreen. There are also some gel variants that offer you protection without clogging your skin. Try the newer powder sunscreen with nano particle technology.

Have happy hair: Hair care should not be ignored during this season. Since the summer's intense UV damage makes the hair dry, frizzy, damaged, getting your hair wet in the rains will further weaken them. So say no to all hair treatments that make use of heat and chemicals. Ironing semi wet or wet hair is a sin.

Work towards healthy hair

- ✤ Coconut oil massage
- ✤ Dry wet hair with low heat
- ✤ Do not brush wet hair
- ✤ Use loose hair accessories
- ✤ Avoid salon treatments—any chemical treatment will harm the strands since the cuticles are open

Monsoon Must Dos

- ✤ Getting wet in the rain is fun but change your clothes as soon as possible. Damp clothes increase the risk of skin infections, especially in body folds.
- ✤ Dry your hair to remove as much moisture as possible. Blows dry your hair gently if needed.
- ✤ Keep wet wipes, moisturizer, face wash, and sunscreen in your purse to keep your skin in great condition.

Supplements to take in monsoon

- ✤ Go high on immune boosters which are your multivitamins.
- ✤ Add anti-inflammatory ingredients to your diet like ginger and turmeric. These ingredients are a major part of our Indian diet.

Monsoon kitchen goodies

- ✤ Papaya face mask—The papain in it removes dead skin layers and tanning.
- ✤ Lemon peel—Turn over half a lemon and use it as a gentle loofah on the face and the body.

- Use a mixture of lemon juice and rice flour paste on face and body to slough off dark, dead skin.
- Apply lemon, curd, and sandalwood powder as mask and then scrub gently to de-tan.

At your skin doctor's

- Most treatments are safe in this season. Concentrate on de-tanning treatments like peels and microdermabrasion.
- Start off laser treatments for skin lightening, tightening, or hair removal.

Winter

A steaming cup of hot chocolate and sitting around the bonfire with friends during the year-end break is all I can think of whenever someone talks about winter. In India, winter means different things in different parts of the country. While people in North India experience really cold temperatures, people in the western and southern regions enjoy pleasant weather. But most people experience dry, dehydrated, rough, sensitive, and chapped skin and lips. Enjoy the chilled wind and water on your face—that can be the best toner ever.

Look and feel of winter skin

- Pale and dry
- Dehydrated and flaky
- Sensitive
- Wrinkled under eyes

- ❖ Chapped lips
- ❖ Dry frizzy hair
- ❖ Prone to breakage
- ❖ Dandruff at its peak

Winter special care

Go overboard with moisturizing: Apply your creamy moisturizer after cleansing your face off all the dead skin and grime as they can act as a barrier against the cream soaking into the skin. Apply moisturizer on damp skin. This not only spreads and hydrates better, but also seals the water on the skin.

Bear the burn: Every patient who comes to me in winter tells me, 'Doc, my skin is so sensitive that any cream that I apply burns my skin,' and so they don't apply any cream at all. What causes the burning is dry and chapped skin, and by not applying cream, they worsen the situation. Even if it burns, don't worry. Apply the cream and let it be. What you could do is spray a mist liberally and apply the cream on top before the effect of the mist dries off. Take plenty of warm fluid intake and healthy amounts of oils in the diet.

Look after your eyes and lips: They lack oil glands and the skin is thin, therefore it dries out and gets wrinkled and chapped. If on any night you do not feel up to skincare, a must-do is eye and lip cream. Since chapping can be a painful condition, give your lips some extra TLC (tender love and care). Exfoliate your lips gently with your finger, then apply a good cold cream, ghee, or lip balm with beeswax. Avoid smacking and licking your lips, as it only aggravates the dryness.

Hands and feet need love: Please make sure the same care that you take with your face is extended to your body as well; especially the exposed parts. Generally go for short bath with warm and not too hot water. Hot water bath is tempting but it also leads to skin's drying. Do not step into a room with heaters immediately after a shower. Pat dry but before that, apply plenty of moisturizer on the damp body. A good but gentle exfoliation and oil indulgence helps. Post oil massage, do not overuse soap. Try a moisturizing body wash instead. Even a 5 minute pre-shower oil massaged on to the body helps in a big way.

Winter must dos

- Move from a foamy face wash to a creamy one and cleanse your face not more than three times a day
- Change liquid remover to a creamy one
- Apply plenty of under eye and lip cream
- Switch from shower gels to shower oils
- Pre bath indulgence with a five minute oil massage
- Oil hair overnight
- Plenty of moisturizer
- Avoid scrubs
- Hydrate
- Use sunscreen

Winter No-No

- ❖ Long, hot baths
- ❖ Avoiding sunscreen
- ❖ Skipping shampoo
- ❖ Petroleum jelly on your lips
- ❖ Licking or smacking your lips

WHY YOU SHOULD AVOID PETROLEUM JELLY FOR YOUR LIPS?

Absolutely no petroleum jelly on your lips! Petroleum jelly acts like a barrier on skin, so if there is moisture on the surface and you have applied the jelly, it stops the moisture from evaporating. Most commonly you use chapstick when your lips are dry and chapped, but the petroleum jelly in the chapstick will not allow the outside moisture to touch your lips, which can dry out your lips further. I am sure you may have noticed that with certain lip-balms, the existing condition gets worse. Therefore, apply plenty of cream like good old Pond's or try ghee. It nourishes the skin instantly. No petroleum jelly. Look for beeswax or shea butter instead.

Supplements for winter

- ❖ Essential fatty acids—Omega 3, 6, 9; codliver oil, fish oil capsules
- ❖ Proteins—whey proteins, simply threptin biscuits, some multivitamins with amino acids
- ❖ Zinc—usually in multivitamin capsules, or with calcium or iron supplements or separately with magnesium

Winter kitchen goodies

- ✤ Honey and banana mask for hydrating skin
- ✤ Milk cream on its own or with sandalwood paste
- ✤ Coconut oil to create a protective barrier on the skin
- ✤ Coconut milk and coconut cream to moisturize your face and body
- ✤ Avoid acidic fruits as mask in winter
- ✤ Fenugreek paste + lemon + coconut milk as a hair mask. Takes care of dry hair and scalp

At your skin doctor's

TO DO

Pampering yourself with hydrating treatments like Hydra facials to bring back lost moisture and stimulate blood flow to the skin.

- ✤ Mesotherapy where non-crosslinked hyaluronic acid is used. This boosts the hydration deep down to the inner layers of the skin and also stimulates collagen. It puts the bounce back into your skin and is an even more long lasting solution. The results are also better.

    Treatments for lips and under eyes to get plumped skin.

TO AVOID

- ✤ Harsh acidic peels and microdermabrasion on sensitive and dry skin

WHAT IS HYALURONIC ACID?

Hyaluronic acid is a super hydrant, i.e. it acts as water to the skin. It stimulates collagen and helps tissue repair—whether applied topically or injected into the layers of the skin. When applied, it may sting a little because of the pH which is acidic but essentially it hydrates the skin. If injected, two forms can be used—the crosslinked and the non-crosslinked form. Because in the natural form hyaluronic acid stays on only for 24 hours, it is degraded by an enzyme present in our body called hyaluronidase. Therefore when injected in the non-crosslinked form, it only increases hydration and stimulates collagen . If you need structural modification and tissue enhancement, like when used as fillers, it is crosslinked and depending on the crosslinking and the molecular size, it stays anywhere between 6 months to 2 years and longer when repeated. This one does not have any species specificity, i.e. you could use the hyaluronic acid on sheep, cows, humans, it does not matter. There is no allergic or any untoward reaction
whatsoever.

In the non-crosslinked form, it is used for treating fine lines, rough and dry skin, loss of skin elasticity, hydration of neck, décolletage, hand skin, and atopic conditions in the folds of the arms. In the crosslinked form, it is used as filler for deep lines, facial enhancement like chin, cheek augmentation, lip contouring, and neck and hand rejuvenation.

Winter care for men

Since guys shave and use aftershave regularly, their skin is more dry and sensitive. If you can, avoid shaving daily.

Before you shave, use hair conditioner on your beard for five minutes to soften the stubble. Use an alcohol or mint-free aftershave.

Do not forget to use moisturizer after shaving.

For more updated information on seasonal skincare, visit my Facebook page (https://www.facebook.com/drrashmiraishetty) or Twitter profile (https://twitter.com/drrashmishetty).

CHAPTER 7

FESTIVE, BRIDAL, AND TRAVEL SKINCARE

THERE'S ALWAYS AN EXCITEMENT when Holi or Diwali is around the corner. It's all about fun, mingling with your friends and family, and eating sweets and fried snacks. But as I said before, what goes inside you shows up externally. Here I have shared some tips on what you should do to keep your skin glowing during the festive season.

Happy Holi, Skin and Hair

Before you step out to join your friends for the festival of colours, here's what you should do:

➢ Massaging your scalp and hair with a coconut-based hair oil is an absolute must. This acts as a barrier and prevents colours from coming in direct contact with hair cuticles and scalp, which means less damage and scalp irritation.

➢ Preferably, tie up your hair before you step out. Leaving you hair open means tangled and damaged

strands. You can wear a fashionable side braid or a
side ponytail. You can also wear a hair-band/scarf
or a bandana around your head to avoid getting
too much chemical-based Holi colours into your
scalp ad hair.

> Do not forget to moisturize your skin well before
you set out to play Holi. This will help in removing
the colour from your skin more easily. Natural
ingredients-based moisturizers like coconut-based
moisturizers are good for your skin. Do not just
moisturize your face, moisturizing your entire
body is equally important.

> Apply a sunscreen since it gets very hot during this
season and all that colour and heat can aggravate
skin damage.

After Holi

> Wash your hair with plain water so that most of
the colour comes off. Then use a mild shampoo. It
is possible for some colour residue to stick to your
scalp. Do not panic! It may take a day or two to
fade away.

> Resist the temptation to wash your hair twice
on the same day. It can make your hair drier. If
you feel your hair is becoming dry, massage the
strands and roots with coconut oil regularly before
shampooing your hair. Since coconut oil is very
light, a single wash with shampoo removes the
unwanted grease very easily.

> A bath immediately after playing Holi is important
so that the colours get off your skin easily. Since
your skin is already exposed to the chemicals from

colours, make sure you do not bathe in water which is too hot as it will irritate your skin even more. Using a foaming body wash to rinse works well. Apply a generous dollop of moisturizer all over your face and body to stave off the irritation that the chemical in the colours can cause.

Bright and beautiful Diwali

Diwali is a time of fun, beauty, and indulgence. It means lots of sweets that you can't resist, even when your well-informed mind is screaming NO. I know all the social responsibility messages that we hear about crackers makes it easier for you to say NO to them, but not too many people put it to practice, do they? So you will still have smoke, toxins, and pollution floating thick in the air for 3 to 5 days after the festival is over.

Then there are the endless pre-Diwali and Diwali parties. So there starts the blow drying, ironing, styling, make up, late nights, and to top it all, the alcohol and may be cigarettes—how these affect your weight, lungs, and liver, let's not even get there. Let me for now just touch the surface, and talk about your skin and hair.

What you need to pay heed to

➢ **Sugar:** It suppresses the activity of our white blood cells and thus makes us more susceptible to colds, flu etc. It also worsens allergies and causes damage because of the breaking down of good proteins, leading to advanced glycation end-products, very aptly abbreviated as AGE. AGE makes the proteins in the collagen and hair stiff and hard;

thus speeding up the process of skin ageing and making hair brittle. As a skin and hair expert, I know that one of the main reasons for wrinkles, deep lines, and sagging skin is AGE. So gorging high sugar foods during Diwali can lead to fine lines and excessive dryness. My suggestion is to be mindful of what you are eating during this time and be aware of what's going into your mouth.

➤ **Smoke:** Smoke and pollution damage hair and skin. You will find your skin dry and scalp irritated or even itchy. Too much exposure can lead to boils/folliculitis, skin rash, and acne exacerbation. You will need to wash your hair and body thoroughly the day after to counteract the damage caused by smoke and ash.

➤ **Excessive make up and styling:** You need to dress up and look pretty on Diwali. This means excessive make up and hair styling products, blow drying, and ironing. Not all this is harmful, but what worsens the situation is when you are too tired to take them all off after the party is over. You might end up missing your night-time skincare regime and cleansing your hair of all the styling products.

➤ **Alcohol and cigarettes:** These worsen the condition of your hair and skin. Alcohol makes the skin flushed and dehydrated with broken capillaries. And cigarettes compromise the blood supply to your skin!

Here's what you must do

➤ Be on a healthy diet always, specially a month before Diwali.

➤ Start oiling your hair with light oils like the ones which are coconut-based.

➤ Avoid too many sweets.

➤ Drink plenty of fluids like water and try to cut down on your alcohol intake.

➤ Remove every trace of make up and apply a good nourishing night cream.

➤ Apply an antioxidant cream which contains vitamin A,C,E, or Q10. Apply it during the day, underneath your sunscreen.

➤ Do not use mousse on hair. If you do, then wash it off at night or the next morning.

➤ Avoid harsh surface chemical treatments during the Diwali month—be it for skin or hair.

➤ Opt for blow drying with low heat since it is better than ironing. Ironing can lead to hair breakage.

➤ Find a little time daily for doing some cardio exercise.

Bridal Advice

As the big day approaches, it's important the bride looks good form head to toe. Right from her skin to her face to her hair, every inch of her body must be perfect.

General tips for hair, body, and skin 3-6 months in advance

❖ First and foremost, consult the right doctor.

❖ Right nutrition and a proper diet are important for beautiful glowing skin.

❖ Supplements rich in protein, calcium, iron, vitamin B3, B6, B12, and antioxidants are very important and help in nourishing the skin.

❖ Weddings can be really stressful and the stress can lead to acne, breakouts, and rashes. For those who cannot handle stress well and want to avoid the above, make sure to apply and also take supplements rich in Vitamin A, C, and E and Coenzyme Q 10.

❖ A daily workout regime which includes yoga and routine exercises is a must. A good workout is not only a great stress buster but also gets the blood rushing, leading to the release of right hormones.

❖ Start off by using the right peels and Medi-Facials for your skin type. It is ideal that you start your skincare routine at least 3 months in advance so any acne and pigmentation have enough time to clear up easily. Skincare is no magic and it takes time to get the best results. It's also a good time to try lasers for any unevenness in your complexion or fractional lasers and micro-needling with radio frequency for old acne pit marks. These may also be used for those stretch marks that you got during your teenage weight loss days. Today, you have an array of gadgets to choose from to make your skin look perfect. If you have dull skin and if you are a 35+ bride then your skin could look great with micro-injections of hyaluronic acid.

- When it comes to your body, make sure you take cream and oil massages and keep your skin exfoliated. Focus on your feet, hands, neck, and décolletage.
- If you are considering laser hair removal, then it is ideal to start it at least 6 months in advance.
- To keep the hair luscious and beautiful, regular oiling, washing, and conditioning every 2-3 days is a must. I'd suggest doing Mesotherapy, a popular treatment that helps in making thin and weak hair strong and thick.

When you have one month to go

- All the above mentioned steps should be followed.
- For tired looking eyes, I recommend under eye filler which will make you look fresh and reduce under eye lines instantly in just one sitting. Lip filler is another popular treatment that helps in plumping your lips slightly which further softens your face, making you look absolutely gorgeous and glamorous. It is not necessary that your lip shape needs to change when you do a slight refreshing of your lips.
- If you suffer from excessive perspiration or hyperhydrosis, then this is the right time to try Botox injections instead of being seen with and ruining your most beautiful outfits with an embarrassing big, wet underarm patch.

1 week before the wedding

❖ Do not start anything new if you have not done it before. Sometimes things can go terribly wrong and you don't want last minute mishaps as there is no time for recovery.

❖ Make sure you indulge in only the mildest peels or microdermabrasion and Medi-Facials.

❖ Everyone has heard of Botox and it's a great way to shape your eyebrows and give you that glamorous arch. Filler, a no down time, very low risk method of non-surgical nose sculpting is also becoming very popular.

❖ Q switched NdYag laser is a safe and good option if you opt for lasers.

❖ Opt for regular, full body hydration, exfoliation, dermabrasion, and peels, and make sure you do not ignore the basics of sunscreen and moisturizer application.

Your SOS kit for the big day

❖ Calandula or Caladryl mixed with very mild steroid application—keep this as an emergency pack in case of a break out or a rash.

❖ Since you're going to apply make up for long hours, keep a hydrating mist with you at all times. It will help you look refreshed.

❖ Keep a derma-shield ointment or petroleum jelly if you're allergic to metal or any fabric or if jewellery doesn't suit your skin.

Honeymoon skincare for brides to be

One important advice I would like to give to all the brides is to maintain your skincare routine even after you are married. Usually, before the wedding you go all out to do the best for your skincare, you go to the best doctor, get the best of everything, pamper your skin like never before for 3-4 months, and once the D-Day happens, its all over all of a sudden.

I have never seen a bride come to me asking for skincare advice post wedding. The next time I see them, is usually when they are panicking with a bad tan or a breakout. So to most of the women who come to me before their wedding for different treatments, I tell them that they need to take care of their skin before the wedding, through the wedding, and post wedding as well.

Make sure you carry on your skincare routine as meticulously as you were doing it before the D-Day.

It might not be possible to go for regular treatments once you are married, as you have so many things to do, so many relatives to meet, before you go for your honeymoon.

So, in advance you should plan with your doctor about your post wedding skincare routine.

Say, for example, if you are not doing a peel every week anymore, you should be doing some appropriate home treatments after the wedding in consultation with your doctor. Depending upon your skin type; there are milder peels that can be used at home.

To continue taking care, also make sure you do not stop the oral supplements that you've been taking.

On your honeymoon, you want to look good 24/7, so you are bound to wear make up most of the time, but no matter how tired or busy you are, do not forget to remove your make up at the end of the day.

Always an emergency kit at hand. A new relationship often gives you a lot of excitement and there are other things like travelling and meeting relatives that can also add on to a lot of stress. Add to it the food you are eating, the sleep you are being deprived of—all this adds extra stress to the skin too. In such a situation you may have breakouts, so an emergency kit with anti-breakout creams is important.

It is also very important to ensure you are getting sufficient rest. Plan your itinerary in such a way that there is enough time for rest.

In a nutshell

- ❖ Don't give up your skincare completely after the wedding.
- ❖ Continue taking oral supplements.
- ❖ Make sure you remove your make up at the end of the day.
- ❖ Keep an emergency kit to deal with sudden breakouts.
- ❖ Get enough rest, so that there's no excessive stress to your body and skin.

On a seaside honeymoon

Depending on which place you are going to, among the most important things to carry in your bag is plenty of sunscreen. Also carry liberal amounts for your favourite hand and body lotion.

Make sure you carry a calamine lotion or any other calming and soothing balm. So, if you are on a seaside trip with a lot of sun exposure on the beach, make sure you apply sunscreen. Wash your skin post the sun exposure and apply the calming lotion it will reduce the chance of inflammation.

On a hill station

If you are on a hill station, cold cream is good for you. Having said that, sunscreen is equally important.

Also do not forget to take care of your lips. You so do not want chapped lips at the end of your honeymoon, so carry a very good lip balm or use plain cold cream.

In a temperate zone

If you are vacationing in a temperate zone where it is very humid, make sure you carry a good face wash that doesn't dry up your skin but takes away excess humidity.

Instead of washing your face twice, do it thrice a day to take out the grime and humidity. It is essential to keep all of your body dry.

Also keep an anti-bacterial powder and cream handy. Take a very mild steroid cream with you, in case you have a reaction or rash and use it as an SOS medication.

Other Dos

Drink enough water so that even if you are drinking a lot of alcohol or eating a lot of junk food, your body remains cleansed. And if you are eating junk food or binging, make sure you take your vitamins and ensure some crucial workouts to keep the body and skin in shape.

It is also important to take care of your hair. If on a beach, oil your hair well or use a sun protection serum. Even plain coconut oil acts as a very good sun protection agent.

Partner's hygiene

You should also be prepared for a beard rash. Make sure your husband is clean-shaven, and if he has a 2-3 day stubble, it should be softened with regular hair conditioner.

Beware of your husband's dandruff as well. Take care of not just your skin and scalp, but also your partner's. The bonding process does not necessarily mean that you share towels and combs.

Leaving on a jet plane

We are 'in' today and 'out' tomorrow! While travelling, the aircraft becomes our second home, where we travel within the country or across countries and continents. Whether it's a long haul flight or a short one, your skin takes a beating. High altitude, higher UV ray exposure, pressurized air conditioners, dehumidified air—all take a toll on your skin. Also during a long haul flight, you are sedentary, therefore you have reduced microcirculation. You tend to drink less water, drink alcohol, eat in excess, and thus so you pack sugar on to an already dry and stressed skin. Alcohol further dehydrates your skin and hair. Therefore you need special care while you are travelling by flight.

1. *Moisturize your skin Moisturize your* face and body liberally before you get on a plane. This will prevent your skin from getting dry to a great extent. If you are worried about the sticky feeling, then try using lotions or moisturizing milk. That gives you the necessary moisture. If you are going to stay in the plane for long, then reapply the moisturizer every once in a while. You can ask for a hot towel, and wipe your face, hands, and feet and reapply the lotion.

2. *Sunscreen is a must especially* if you are flying during the day, more so if you choose a window seat or if you are a pilot. Make sure you have applied a good amount of sunscreen on all the exposed parts and not just the face. This keeps you away from burning sensation, redness, and tanning. Remember, whatever the SPF, it is wise to apply sunscreen every 2 to 3 hours. This is important when you know the intensity of UV rays is really harsh because of the altitude.

3. *Get liberal with thermal water spray* which will keep your skin's hydration levels balanced. The good news is that you can even spray it over make up without the fear of getting your make up ruined. Spray it even before you apply your moisturizer so that your skin stays plump and supple.

4. *Skin around your eye and lip* has no oil glands and are stretched thin (as I mentioned in an earlier section), so make sure you take extra care of these areas. Always keep a really good under eye cream handy and a lip balm, which you can repeatedly apply. I am not a fan of petroleum jelly, so I suggest you use a good lip balm instead.

5. *Make sure you have conditioned your hair* or you can use light oils like coconut based ones and tie your hair up if you are not flying for a special occasion. If not, you could tie a scarf around your hair. This will prevent the strands from drying out and getting static and frizzy.

6. *Have plenty of water and fruits*. Avoid alcohol and too much caffeine.

7. *Get up and stretch often*; it increases peripheral blood flow and avoids venous stagnation. This way you will not get the swelling you may get otherwise. You can also avoid other medical complications due to sluggish circulation.

Make a little kit that you can carry along

You can either ask your doctor to give you sample-size packs of your routine skincare products or you can buy small plastic bottles and jars easily available at beauty and health stores and put in a little of the products in them to carry with you in flight.

Your kit should contain a facial mist, moisturizing milk or lotion, under eye cream, lip butter with shea or beeswax, sunscreen, and wet wipes.

Travel care

If you are packing your bags for an exotic travel destination, make sure your skin is prepared to face the environmental onslaught of that place. Holiday getaways can be refreshing for the body and soul and de-stress your mind, but when you loosen your knots and blast out on a new destination, you often tend to ignore the needs of your skin. The harsh sun of on island can leave sunburns and the dry winds of a mountain getaway can cause dryness. So, as you step out on a vacation, do not forget the needs of your skin. You certainly do not want dull, dry, and patchy skin when you return from the holiday.

- Make sure you **moisturize** and hydrate your skin in advance of your travel plans. When we travel, we often get busy in other details and forget our skincare regime. Moisturize your skin and hair at least a week in advance—coconut oil is a good option for a skin and hair massage that will deeply hydrate the body and scalp. Some hydrating cosmetic procedures and hydrating facials can be beneficial, so is a session with hyaluronic acid based dermal fillers like Juvederm. This will provide you enough deep hydration to last for a few months.

- It is always good to take **oral supplements** rich in vitamins and Omega-3 for your skin. If you are going on a long haul, carry the supplements with you and consume them daily. Vitamins have powerful antioxidants that prevent free radical damage.

- If you are heading to a sunny destination, it would be good to take a Botox shot for your frown lines a week in advance because sun glare accentuates them and you do not want to return from the vacation with accentuated frown lines. This will also make you look fresh and relaxed at the holiday.

- If you have to spend the day out in the open, you should take care of removing the layer of dust and pollution or even bacteria that settles on top of your skin. Make sure to carry a face wash and a moisturizer in your handbag and keep washing your face and applying the lotion 2-3 times a day. Also carry quality wet face wipes that can come to your help in case you do not have clean water. When travelling, you want to look good 24/7, so you are bound to wear make up most of the time. But no matter however tired or busy you are, do not forget to remove your make up at the end of the day.

- If you are on a holiday, you are bound to spend most of the time outdoors even if it is a humid and hot destination. Excessive sweating in such situations can be a problem. It would help if you undertake a Botox procedure to cut down on underarm sweating. We all know how excessive sweating on the palms can be such a social and professional embarrassment. When administered under the arm, Botox can control the sweat glands and prevent sweating that can cause discomfort, patches on the clothes, and body odour.

- Carry an emergency kit. Travelling, whether for leisure or meeting relatives, can give you a lot of stress. Add to it the food you are eating and the sleep you are being deprived of which extra stress to the skin too. In such a situation you may have breakouts, so an emergency kit with anti-breakout applicants is important.

- It is also very important to ensure you are taking sufficient rest. Plan your itinerary in such a way that there is enough time for rest.

- Don't forget to carry a good protective pair of sunglasses on a summer destination. They are vital to protect the eyes against the glare of the sun and also the delicate skin around the eyes. Better go for a UV protection offering product.

- Always carry a hand sanitizer, because we keep touching our faces with hands and you certainly do not want to infect your face skin.

- If your face sweats a lot, carry a spring water mist and keep spraying on your face and wiping with a tissue to keep yourself fresh. Also, do not keep reusing your hand towel.

- Drink enough water so that even if you are drinking a lot of alcohol or consuming junk food, your body should be cleansed. And if you are eating junk food or binging, make sure you take your vitamins and take out time for some crucial workouts to keep the body and skin fine.

- It is important to take care of your hair too. If on a beach, oil your hair well or use a **sun protection serum**. Even **plain coconut oil** acts as a very good sun protection agent.

Your skincare will also depend on the type of destination you are heading to.

On a sea side vacation

Depending on which place you are going to, among the most important things to carry in your bag is **plenty of sunscreen**. Carry liberal amounts for your hand and body as well. While you are under the sun directly, the reflection from the sea accentuates the glare. So, you not just need sunscreen, you need a thick layer of sunscreen for protection.

Also make sure you carry a calamine lotion or any other calming and soothing balm. Once back from the sea, bathe yourself in cold water to soothe and calm the skin and also to remove salt from your skin surface that can cause irritation. On a seaside, salt is not just in the water, but also in the air. Post washing, apply the calming lotion for it reduces chances of inflammation.

On a hill station

If you are on a hill station, **cold cream** is good for you. Having said that, sunscreen is equally important.

Also do not forget your lips. You so not want chapped lips at the end of your vacation, so do carry a very good **lip balm** or use plain cold cream for the purpose. Also apply cream liberally around your eyes and lips. In winters, it's also advisable to carry a cleanser with glycolic acid. VIVITE can be a good option. Work on your skin for 2-3 minutes in small circular motions which will loosen the dead skin on top and make it more receptive to the moisturizer.

In a temperate zone

If you are vacationing in a temperate zone where it is very humid, make sure you carry **a good face wash** that does not dry up your skin but takes away excess humidity.

Instead of washing twice, do it thrice a day to remove grime and humidity. Another important prerequisite is to keep your body dry.

Also keep an anti-bacterial powder and cream handy. Take a **very mild steroid cream** with you, in case you have a reaction or rash and use it as an SOS medication.

PART II
Cheat the Clock

CHAPTER 8
SKINCARE ESSENTIALS

THERE IS SO MUCH conflicting information out there about how to retain your skin's youthfulness which can often leave you confused and make you pick up products that may or may not work. I have seen so many women who come to me quite disillusioned about the products they use, or even about the whole concept of proper skincare. In most cases, I see that there are minor deviations that can be set right with just a bit of tweaking. This chapter will tell you what all you need to have in your skincare bag.

Getting the tools right first

As you begin on the path of getting skin that is smooth, supple, and glowing from within, you need to start with the right tools. They form the basis of your skincare routine, ensuring that your creams and potions work effectively to keep your skin soft and supple.

Cotton pads: You will need them to wipe away your make up and for your cleansing lotion. But make sure that the cotton pads are smooth and without any fibre sticking out so they don't irritate the skin.

A piece of muslin: Instead of using regular Turkish towels to wipe your face after a wash, use a soft muslin cloth. It is gentler and absorbs water faster without hurting the skin. Dab it on the skin to soak up excess water. Avoid rubbing—it can seriously harm your skin and cause pigmentation.

Cool gel packs: They are easily available at beauty stores and pharmacies. Pick up one for the eyes and face. They are instant soothers and can tone up tired skin effectively. Stock them in the fridge. They are instant skin pick-me-ups.

Shower cap or cling film: A shower cap makes an interesting thermal mask to help creams penetrate deeper into your skin and hair. You can simply cut a little hole for the nose area and then wear it after applying some deep moisturizing creams. This works well for highly dehydrated and dry skin. You can even try this with cling films that you use to pack food in.

Spatula: It is always a good idea to have a spatula in case you need to dig into a pot of cream, apply a mask, or take off a creamy mask. Remember to keep the spatula clean after using it. Easy way is to get some ice cream sticks.

Tweezer: I consider the tweezer as one of the best tools for instant beautification, not just to pull out those extra hairs on the chin or upper lip, but to even keep your eyebrows in top shape.

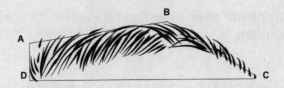

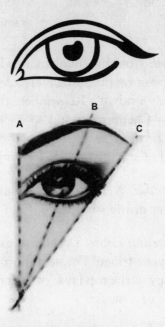

Beauty potions from your kitchen

Arundhathi Rai, a naturopath, believes that no skincare regime is complete without a dose of the 'naturals'. But you don't really need to scour exotic food stores to pick up imported herbs or extracts. Just head to your local supermarket and stock up on the regular items that you can use for a healthy diet and apply on your skin as well. Arundhathi says that whatever fruit remains on your fruit platter after a meal, put it on your face instead of discarding it.

> 'Ever since I've understood the meaning of beauty and skincare, I have always been using natural products, including home remedies.'
>
> Yami Gautam, Actress

Coconut oil: Contains linolenic acid and is of straight chain composition (meaning molecules in this compound are aligned straight. Remember the pentagons and octagons in Chemistry?) and so it penetrates into your skin and hair more easily as compared to the rest of the oils instead of staying on top, forming a barrier.

Coconut milk: A great hair conditioner/masque for soothing dry brittle strands.

Coconut cream: Grate a coconut, extract its milk, and let it sit in your fridge. The next morning, after the water settles, take out the top layer of the cream and use it as a moisturizer or a mask.

Coriander seeds: It can be a great eye soother. Soak the seeds overnight and then put it into little gauze bags. Put these over your tired eyes; they will look bright in no time.

Cucumber: Soothes tired eyes and minimizes dark circles.

Eggs: It is a skin and hair nourisher. An egg mask lifts and hydrates the skin instantly, but remember to put in some essential oil (jojoba if the skin is dry, lavender if the skin is flushed, or basil if acne prone) to mask the smell.

Fenugreek seeds: Soak the seeds overnight and grind it into a paste the next day. It makes for an excellent hair pack.

Gram flour: If you are indoors most of the times and your skin does not have any particular issue, gram flour acts as a great replacement for soap and can be used as a gentle skin exfoliator.

Honey: Gives you dewy, glowing skin in an instant. Superb hydrant.

Lemon: Give your skin a big dose of vitamin C. It is a natural skin lightening agent and acid peel.

Masoor dal (red lentils): Ideal for using as a scrub or mask to treat dry skin.

Milk: Soothes sun-irritated skin. Milk can also be used as a medium to make any paste or mask, like when you use it while rubbing sandalwood on a rough stone to make a paste.

Oatmeal/Rice powder: The ideal body/face scrub to treat dry, itchy skin.

Potatoes: The juice of potatoes can fight pigmentation.

Sandalwood paste: Get a piece of the sandalwood and rub it on a wet stone with milk or water. The paste helps fight acne and pigmentation and calms irritated skin.

Strawberries/Grapes: Give your skin a dose of antioxidants and vitamin C with these.

Sugar: Great skin polisher.

Papaya/Green Apple: Both are rich in enzymes. They loosen dead skin by gently exfoliating it and give your skin a nice glow.

Tomatoes: Lighten acne scars, pigmentation, and excessive oiliness by applying this.

Tender coconut water: Dab some on your face to heal dehydrated skin and scars.

Tulsi (Indian/Holy Basil): Treat acne and skin irritation.

Turmeric: A natural antiseptic and best anti-inflammatory ingredient. You will find its powder in every Indian kitchen. Get fresh turmeric root and rub it on wet stone to make a paste.

Used teabags: Reduce puffy eyes with these.

Wheatgrass: It is a shot of pure health when freshly extracted and gives a good dose of iron.

Yogurt: When consumed, the good bacteria not only helps your tummy, it also brightens tired skin. When applied, the acid in the curd helps in lightening and hydrating the skin.

CHAPTER 9

NECESSARY NUTRIENTS

As a doctor I know the importance of nutrients for the skin. However, when there are experts in specific fields who can provide more in-depth information, I'd rather you get it straight from them. My expert friends are going to give you gyan on nutrition and some fantastic anti-ageing recipes. However, I want to tell you from a doctor's perspective that there area few things you must do.

Nutrients for Skin and Hair

As I have already said in the earlier chapters, what you put in your mouth shows on your skin and hair. So here's a list of diet essentials that you have to ensure gets on your plate every day.

Macronutrients

These are the three food essentials—proteins, carbohydrates, and fats—that our body needs in large quantities to stay healthy. They support the cell structure of our body.

PROTEINS: Proteins are fundamental components of all living cells and include many substances such as enzymes, hormones, and antibodies that are necessary for the proper functioning of an organism. Protein is the key element in our skin and hair make up. They are essential in the diet of animals for the growth and repair of tissues. Your body converts standard proteins that you eat into keratin protein to make up your hair, skin, and nails. Ensuring that you include one source of protein in every meal of your day will help hair growth. That said, the amount of protein required depends on the age and ideal body weight of an individual.

BEST FOOD SOURCES: Eggs, lean cuts of chicken, oily fish, lentils, soy or tofu, and spirulina.

CARBOHYDRATES: Despite varying reports about carbohydrates, it is an essential part of your diet. Carbohydrates are a group of organic compounds that include sugar, starch, cellulos, and gum and they serve as a major energy source for us. Carbohydrates sourced from plants give you fibre that regulate your cholesterol and blood sugar. Fibre also helps in eliminating toxins from our body and in better absorption of the nutrients. However, you have to make sure you get your carbohydrates from plant sources and whole grains, and avoid 'white' or 'refined' carbohydrates.

BEST FOOD SOURCES: Whole grains, unpolished dals, oats, brown rice, beans like rajma, carrots, spinach etc.

FATS: Among the macronutrients, fat is essential for supple skin texture and glow. The micronutrients that are essential for skin protection require fat as a medium for absorption. Essential Fatty Acids (EFA) is another nutrient that cannot be made by our body and is required to be consumed through our diet. EFAs are responsible for skin repair, moisture content, and overall flexibility. Dry, inflamed skin or skin that suffers from the frequent appearance of whiteheads or blackheads can benefit from supplementing with EFAs. EFAs are essential to grow hair. About 3% of the hair shaft is made up of these fatty acids. There are two types of EFAs—Omega-3 and Omega-6—that we need to keep our skin and hair healthy.

Omega-6 fatty acids promote hair growth and support skin cell renewal, while Omega-3 fatty acids moisturize your skin and hair follicles for long, radiant hair and a smooth complexion. Omega-3s are also found in cell membranes in the skin of your scalp, and in the natural oils that keep your scalp and hair hydrated. Chances are that you already consume enough Omega-6 fatty acids, so focus on increasing your Omega-3 fatty acid intake. For healthy adults, a combined daily total of 500 milligrams (mg) EPA + DHA is recommended either from diet (i.e. oily fish) or supplements. While having fish for dinner is one way to get EPA and DHA, most people don't eat the suggested two to three servings of oily fish per week to reap the benefits of these powerful nutrients.

BEST FOOD SOURCES: Walnuts, flax seeds, chia seeds, peanut butter, fatty fish like salmon, cod liver oil supplements, and primrose oil supplements.

Easy sources of EFA

GHEE: Among the fats used in our diet, ghee is rich in antioxidants and acts as an aid in the absorption of vitamins and minerals from other foods, serving to strengthen the immune system and prevent skin damage.

FISH OIL SUPPLEMENTS: You can have these to get your daily requirement of Omega-3s. When you are out shopping for them, be sure to determine how much Omega-3s are provided per serving. The average 1000 mg fish oil softgel typically provides around 300 mg of Omega-3s (even less of the important EPA and DHA), so in order to meet the 500 mg intake guidelines, a minimum of two softgels would be necessary.

Micronutrients

They are essential elements that our body needs to function and regenerate effectively. The main function of micronutrients is to enable many chemical reactions to occur in our body which lead to growth and repair of skin and hair cells. However they are needed in small amounts.

ANTIOXIDANTS: Vitamin A, C, and E are essential micronutrients that prevent any free radical damage to the skin. They are very powerful antioxidants which ensure the skin cells are safe from harm caused by oxidation.

VITAMIN A: Stimulates cell turnover. It also helps to produce healthy sebum.

BEST FOOD SOURCES: Sweet potato, carrot, spinach, peaches, and cod liver oil.

RECOMMENDED DAILY INTAKE: One medium-sized carrot with 1 bowl of salad with greens everyday should give you the required amount of vitamin A

VITAMIN C: Vitamin C helps you grow strong skin, hair, and nails, and fight sun damage.

BEST FOOD SOURCES: Blueberries, gooseberries, strawberries, and oranges.

RECOMMENDED DAILY INTAKE: A cup each of blueberries and strawberries can help you get your required amount of vitamin C.

VITAMIN E: Adds moisture to your cells, and makes skin and hair shine with health. It all works to stabilize the cell membranes. This vitamin also works with the mineral selenium to ward off attacks on the cells in your follicles.

BEST FOOD SOURCES: Sunflower seeds, almonds, papaya, bell peppers.

RECOMMENDED DAILY INTAKE: A quarter cup of sunflower seeds along with 20 almonds in a day can make up for the required amount of vitamin E. Recommended daily intake is 15mg per day.

VITAMIN B6: Several small-scale clinical studies have shown positive results with vitamin B6 as a hair growth agent. Vitamin B6 does a number of things in the body that aids the overall health of the hair, ranging from boosting the immune system to aiding in the formation of red blood cells.

BEST FOOD SOURCES: Tuna fish, lean cuts of poultry, potatoes, sunflower seeds, and bananas.

RECOMMENDED DAILY INTAKE: 1.3 mg/day for adults.

VITAMIN B12: In regards to human hair, the hair follicles require vitamin B12 in order to properly replicate and if they are not able to, they cannot grow hair effectively. The follicles also require oxygen just like the rest of your body and if there is a shortage of B12, it prevents red blood cells from being properly made in the bone marrow, and the follicles don't receive proper nutrients resulting in hair loss and a slowing down of hair growth. Vegetarians and specifically vegans will require vitamin B12 supplementation.

BEST FOOD SOURCES: Oily fish, lean cuts of meat, yogurt.

RECOMMENDED DAILY INTAKE: 2-3ug/day for adults.

BIOTIN: Biotin is a vitamin that is needed by our body for the metabolism of various nutrients and the establishment of a number of hormones and enzymes. This substance is needed to support a number of biochemical reactions, including the formation of antibodies. Biotin plays a role in the formation of hormones and enzymes in the body. This vitamin is required for the metabolism of carbohydrates, fats, and proteins and it is very important for hair's maintenance and prevention of hair loss.

BEST FOOD SOURCES: Eggs, Swiss chard, liver, almonds, and walnuts.

RECOMMENDED DAILY INTAKE: 35-70 ug per day.

Essential minerals

They are needed by the body to strengthen the skin and hair cells and improve metabolism.

IRON: Iron is especially important; because it helps cells carry oxygen to your skin and hair structure. If there is too little iron (anaemia) women particularly experience hair loss and sallow skin. The body does not absorb the kind of iron generally found in some vegetables and grains as efficiently as it does in case of animal sources of iron. Thus, vegetarians need to increase these allowances by 1.8 times.

BEST FOOD SOURCES: Spinach, soy beans, tofu, liver, meat, and eggs

RECOMMENDED DAILY INTAKE: For adults, the dosage is 8mg per day. Recommended daily intake for women will vary and dependeds on their menopausal or pregnancy status.The maximum intake limit from all sources is 45 mg per day.

ZINC: It is important for normal cell growth. Zinc deficiency weakens the cells, which can result in lesions on the skin. This nutrient also controls the oil production and reduces chances of ageing. Recommended daily intake for adult men is 11mg per day and for adult women it is 8mg per day.

Best food sources: Oysters, pumpkin seeds, sesame seeds, and oats.

Recommended daily intake: 1-2 ounces of oysters can make up for 100% of the daily requirement; vegetarians necessarily may need an oral supplement along with ¼ cup of pumpkin and sesame seeds.

SELENIUM: This nutrient is essential to maintain skin elasticity. One of the most important functions of selenium is as a component of glutathione peroxidase, an enzyme necessary for the antioxidant function of glutathione. Glutathione is one of the major antioxidants in the body that protects against cellular damage from the free radicals that cause inflammation, ageing, and skin cancer. In fact, many scientists support the theory that selenium in the diet protects against skin cancer. Selenium also plays a significant role in acne severity.

Best food sources: Brazil nuts, shellfish, wheat bran.

Recommended daily intake: Just two Brazil nuts a day will give you the 200 micrograms necessary for an adequate intake.

FOLIC ACID: Folic acid plays an important role in repair of damaged hair and in healthy hair growth.

Best food sources: Nuts, soybean, or soymilk.

Recommended daily intake: 400–1000ug/day for adults.

COPPER: Copper is essential for the proper functioning of the body, including healthy hair growth. An inadequate intake of copper can cause hair loss and thinning hair. Copper is also believed to intensify hair colour and delay greying of hair.

BEST FOOD SOURCES: Cocoa powder, dark chocolate, cremini mushrooms, black sesame seeds, and lobster.

RECOMMENDED DAILY INTAKE: 2mg per day.

Some of the supplements that you can take on a daily basis to improve your total health and skin and hair are antioxidant pills, a good multivitamin, a fish oil capsule to get your dose of Omega-3, evening primrose oil, vitamin E, and calcium. After a week, if levels are low then add iron and vitamins D3 and B12 as well.

Don't shy away from supplements because even if you follow a healthy diet, the quantity may not be enough for the necessary amount of essential minerals you may need in a day. A great diet plus some supplements are your secret to good skin and hair.

CHAPTER 10

COMPONENTS OF YOUR SKINCARE REGIME

WHATEVER YOUR SKIN GOAL is, you have to understand that it cannot be achieved in a day. You have to have the discipline to practice a daily skincare regime to see any real results. Now let's talk about the skincare products you may need on a daily basis for your regime.

Step 1: Cleansing

In your cleansing routine, depending on your lifestyle or the necessity of your skin, you would need a make up remover, a cream cleanser or a gel cleanser, and a face wash. The whole process can be divided into three steps.

Make up remover

There are different kinds of make up removal products available in the market. Some are oil-based and can lather up to act like a face wash when applied with water. So you have it all out at one go as such a product takes away the oil soluble make up and emulsifies the rest of it. You could just wash it off and remove it. It is a great product if you are one of those who don't like too many steps in their cleansing process. But if you've applied heavy make up, you may need a separate creamy type make up remover if you are just using a face wash to emulsify the pigment in the coloured make up.

Cleanser

Choose a lotion if you have dry or sensitive skin. Work on your skin moving your fingers in small circular movements and then wipe it off with wet cotton. If you pick a liquid, watery cleanser, then soak a cotton ball and wipe your skin clean with it. Repeat with a fresh cotton pad till your face becomes clean. If your skin is very oily, you could use cleansers which are specially meant for oily skin. It acts more like a toner and you should use it after a face wash.

Face Wash

You'll be surprised how much can be achieved by just choosing the right face wash. Since there are so many face washes available these days with active ingredients, you need to know which one is best suited for your skin type.

> ➤ If you have a very oily skin which is acne prone, choose a face wash with salicylic acid or benzoyl peroxide. If it's just oily, then look for a face wash with neem or tea tree oil with witch hazel in it. There are some really nice face washes in the

market that remove the excess oil without leaving your skin too dry.

➢ If your skin is just about normal, there are wonderful face washes which take off the dirt and grime from your face. Do not look for face washes that list specific ingredients as they might be harsh/irritating or too hydrating for an otherwise normal skin. So go for a strawberry/blackberry/orange flavour. All you want is a fresh face devoid of make up grime.

➢ If your skin is dry, there are creamy washes that clean the skin but retain the moisture.

➢ If your skin looks dull then try a face wash with small exfoliating granules that have a gentle scrubbing action.

➢ If your skin is dull and pigmented, there are face washes with glycolic acid that helps lighten your skin.

As you age, your skin only gets dryer. So make sure you choose a face wash that is more creamy, gentle, and contains fine granules to double up as a scrub. But again you could be 50 with oily skin, so there are always exceptions.

Step 2: Moisturizing

Day Cream

Day creams usually contain sunscreen as the most important ingredient. But you can look for something extra in this. If you can manage to get a cream with pore-refining or oil-soaking (calamine, koline, fuller's earth, volcanic mud) properties along with antioxidants, that would be a great combination to have.

Night Cream

I am sure none of us want to go through a rigorous skincare procedure at night after you come back from work. You are tired; you have to finish your chores at home; so you just have enough strength to do that ONE thing—cleanse your face and then immediately use a night cream. The night cream has to have higher moisture content and be creamier than your day cream. Pick one with skin lightening or anti-ageing actives, since your skin is most receptive at night. You can deal with your skin issues with a good treatment-based night cream like acne prescription creams, skin lightening creams that work on particular areas like the cheek, anti-wrinkle cream, with say retin A, that work on special areas, or simply a cream rich in ceramides if your skin is super dry .

Serum

Most of us think that serum is a super concentrate. However, serums are just active ingredients in a different medium. They are more suited for oily skin types. They also work when you have more than one skin goal to achieve. This means that if you want to use skin lightening or antioxidant in the day time when you have to use a sunscreen, it is a really good idea to use those actives in a serum form first and then apply sunscreen on top.

Mist/thermal spring water spray

The spring water spray, as the name suggests, is sourced from special springs. It is rich in minerals that soothe and soften the skin. A couple of spritzes on your face on a dry, hot day can instantly hydrate your skin and freshen you up as well. It is good for calming inflamed skin. You can get them at a chemist or beauty store. Use them on bare skin, over moisturizer, over sunscreen, or over make up, and your skin will thank you for it.

As you progress in age, you may need heavier creams (if you have dry skin—one with less fat beneath the skin) or then lighter ones (to keep up with hydration if you have oily skin and acne issues) with intense hydration and active ingredients to plump your skin and pep up skin turnover, thus also stimulating collagen. You also have the luxury of layering various portions as your skin now not only needs more, it can also handle more in terms of added moisture and protection.

Aftershave lotion or aftershave balm?

Men who shave on a daily basis almost always use an aftershave product. These are now available in two major forms—a balm or a lotion. Aftershaves act as antiseptic agents that protect skin from infections that can be caused due to minute cuts in the skin during shaving. It is important that you use it immediately after shaving (try to shave directly after taking your shower so that the cuticles are soft). Depending on your skin condition, you can either choose a balm, which is a creamier version, or a lotion which very light textured.

Toners—the most confused term

Earlier toners were considered an important part of one's skincare regime, so most brands had toners. But ever since newer skincare brands introduced face washes and all-in-one cleanser creams in the market, the toner as a product was forgotten. However, I feel toner is a misunderstood product because when you say toner, people think of a skin tightener or a pore shrinking product or a deep cleanser. It really depends on the ingredients that the toner has. Most toners available today actually remove excess oil from the face, and since they have a 'minty' property to them, they also seemingly shrink the pores a bit.

Step 3: Sun protection

The one question I get asked most frequently is, 'Do I really have to apply sunscreen?' My answer is yes, you need to apply sunscreen all the time. For those who just want one single cream—sunscreen is a must. And then you could layer your make up on top of it. Sunscreen is one of the most important skincare products you need to use.

You must remember, we are not trying to protect ourselves from just visible light but the ultraviolet rays of the sun like UV A, B, and C. While UVC hardly reaches us, it is UVA and UVB that you have to be very careful of. UVA penetrates deep and passes through everything including your glass window panes. Therefore, it is very important to apply sunscreen—whether you are indoors or out in the sun or even if the weather is cloudy.

The skin and UV rays

As mentioned before, we need to be careful of both UVA and UVB rays of the sun. The range for UVB is 290 to 320 nanometer, and UVA is 320 to 400 nanometer. Both equally affect the skin.

UVB radiation penetrates the epidermal or outer layer of the skin. It damages DNA in this layer and causes other changes in skin cells. This ultimately may result in the signs of photoageing. Over time, pre-cancers and skin cancers may develop.

UVA radiation, while also damaging the epidermis, penetrates deeper into the skin to the level of the dermis. UVA not only harms epidermal cells, it also damages collagen and elastin, which make up the structure of the dermis and keep the skin resilient. Blood vessels can also be harmed.

Photoageing and what to do

Photoageing is the premature ageing of the skin caused by repeated exposure to ultraviolet radiation (UV) primarily from the sun, but also from artificial UV sources. Photoageing is different from chronological ageing, as the damaging effects are that of UV rays of the sun.

- Alters the normal structures of the skin.
- Vascular damage: The deeper veins become thick and more noticeable under the skin.
- The superficial fine capillaries walls become thin which show as broken capillaries on your skin.
- Increase in number of inflammatory infiltrates which makes your skin sensitive on top.

❖ Causes cell mutations caused by UV. This results in premature ageing, the formation of actinic keratoses or pre-cancers, and skin cancer.

Knowing what to look for in a bottle of sunscreen is very important since the market is cluttered with sunscreen products. You should focus on SPF (Sun Protection Factor) and TPI (Tan Protection Index). A sunscreen with SPF 20 to 50 is more than enough to get almost 98% protection. Anything more adds around 0.5%. So even if you are using a product with SPF 100, your protection won't be a lot different. More SPF does not mean longer protection, it only means more grease and heavy chemical ingredients for just 0.5% extra protection. Generally speaking, 1 SPF gives you 10 minutes of protection under the sun. So go ahead, do the calculation, and choose your sun protection accordingly. But do remember to reapply your sunscreen twice or thrice during the sun up hours.

SPF, however, only means that you will burn less and therefore develop lesser pigmentation. But the actual anti-ageing defence happens from UVA protection. This you can see from the + (plus) sign on the bottle. You can also look for the term 'broad spectrum' which means a sunscreen that protects you from the full spectrum of ultra violet rays—UV A, UV B. Additionally, look for photostability of the ingredient, which means how long they remain active under harsh sunlight. Your sun protection cream may have additional ingredients like pretochopherol and other protective antioxidants.

What adds on most to your chronological age is photoageing, so make sunscreen your skin's best friend.

Your degree of photoageing depends on the person and the type of skin you have. Sun exposure over the years without skin protection can result in visible signs of photoageing. Your skin type and the amount of unprotected sun exposure you get will determine your risk. Those who spend a lot of time in the sun because of outdoor work or recreation also fall into the high risk group. Darker skinned people show fewer signs of obvious photoageing, although the skin can become mottled and there may be some wrinkling.

Go on a skincare fast

Do not overdo things on your skin. It's important to give your skin a break once in a while. Just like the way you fast for your body and for good health, do it once in a while for your skin too. Our elders would keep fasts in the name of religious rituals since they knew that fasting once in a month or fortnight gave us definite health benefits, made us more energetic, and cleansed us from inside. Similarly, your skin also needs to go on a fast. So it's important that you stop using all the products for a night probably and just let the skin be. You can do that once in a while, and see your skin breathe.

MORE IS NOT ALWAYS GOOD

It is not true that:

- ❖ The more you pay, the better the outcome of your cream.
- ❖ Applying more products is always beneficial.
- ❖ Using more means quicker results.

Decoding the Texture

- ❖ Creams: Usually contain 2 phases—oil phase and water phase. 50-80% by weight of cream has water as the primary component; 15-30% oil, and 6-15% emulsifiers. A typical cold cream is mainly water in oil emulsion. This emulsion contains around 55% mineral oil and 12% beeswax and other ingredients.

- ❖ Serums: Formulation which is light, penetrates rapidly, has concentrated actives.

- ❖ Lotions: Cleansing creams and lotions are usually detergent-based or emulsified oil systems that are designed primarily for removal of surface oil. Lotions usually contain 15-50% oil with limited quantities of waxy materials.

Decoding your skincare regime

There are a lot of times when patients come to me with no particular concern as such but just to get their routine right. I am often asked, 'Doc, what are the products you think I should use?' To this my reply is,'If you love the product you have been using and it makes your skin feel perfect, say maybe a sunscreen whose consistency you love, then I don't think there is any reason for you change your brand or the product. If something has suited you so well, you can stick to it for now.'All I then do is play with some actives in terms of correction, if any, and readjust the regime a bit.

The next thing you need to know is how much of your product should you apply, irrespective of what you buy. You could buy the most expensive skincare product on earth or you could buy a tube worth 100 rupees from a medical store which probably has the same ingredients in it as the expensive product, but the results on the skin will depend on how effectively you apply it.

1. How to apply

Do not rub the cream/ lotion on to your palms and then on your face! That is a big no no. Take a bit on your fingertip and then apply it on your skin. After this, gently spread it across your face with just two fingers. I am often asked about how much of any skincare product really permeates our skin. You must know that the external layer of the skin, the epidermis, is technically a dead skin layer which is made of keratin, a protein that tightly adheres to each other. Therefore, it is impossible for any external thing to permeate your skin unless the molecule is of a special size or has some important ingredients which can take the heavier molecules along with it inside. So it's important for us to first:

- ❖ Cleanse the skin so that the oil of the skin is out of the way and it doesn't block the creams.
- ❖ Exfoliate once in a while to make sure that the dead skin is gone. You can go to your skin doctor for chemical peeling or hydra peeling to remove the top dead layer.

2. How much to apply

How much of a particular product you should apply depends on the skin issue that you are dealing with. For example, if the skin is super dry and you are looking for a moisturizer, I would then say definitely douche your skin with enough quantity of the product and after 2-3 hours, you will see that it makes a lot of difference.

But if you are using an active ingredient, like say for acne or for pigmentation or for any specific condition on your skin, then using a lot might further irritate or sometimes make it worse. Start off with a very thin layer, feathering it into your sensitive areas. If your product has active ingredients like acids, then always remember that less is good to start with.

3. When to apply

Use anti -ageing/skin lightening treatment products usually at night. Sunscreens in the sun up hours. Never mind if you are indoors or whether it is a cloudy, rainy, or a windy day.

4. How long to keep it on your skin

Some overnight, some for long hours, and some for just a couple of hours, depending upon your skin doctor's instructions. However, sunscreens have to be reapplied every 4 hours. Ask your doctor these questions when you consult him/her.

By and large, if you keep any product for 2 hours to start with, it will give you an idea about how strong it is, or how well your skin takes it. You will know whether keeping it on for longer makes your skin go red, or too dry, or itchy. You will know all this after keeping it on for two hours for the first time and then removing it. Once your skin settles with the product, you could increase it to overnight application. However, if you are using something more nourishing or replenishing like vitamin creams, antioxidants, or simply moisturizers, then go ahead and be liberal and keep it as long as you want to.

WHEN YOU APPLY A CREAM, SERUM, OR LOTION (CLEANSER, SUNSCREEN, OR NIGHT CREAM), DO IT ON YOUR FACE WITH A FINGER AND WITH TWO FLAT FINGERS, SPREAD THE CREAM ALL OVER WITH FIRM STROKES.

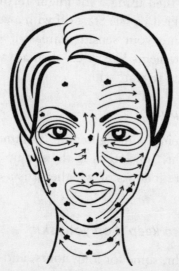

Maximise your potion

The most common question asked in any skincare talk that I have given so far is in which order should one apply one's skincare creams. There's a perpetual confusion as to sunscreen first or sunscreen last and when does the serum go on. So let me try and make it easy for you.

In the right order

> Corrective or a therapeutic agent goes first i.e. right on your skin. It could be anti-ageing, anti-acne, anti-pigmentation—any one of these.

> Nourisher comes next, and it could be a cream or any form of hydrant.
> The protectant—sunscreen—goes on top.
> Coloured make up tops it all.

The right delivery medium

- Serums and gels go first.
- Creams and lotions go next.
- Oils, silicones, and petroleum jellies go on top. Because once you apply these nothing else ever penetrates.

How to get a clean face

- *Remove make up first:* Intensely pigmented make up—which is usually the eye, eyebrow, and lip make up—needs to be removed first. After you have gotten rid of this, use the make up remover for the rest of your face and neck. Always use separate cotton for each area. Using wrong strokes and harsh product to remove the eye make up may lead to loosening of skin in that area, so do it carefully. This can burst the tiny capillaries and cause blood cells to get accumulated which make the eye and under eye area look dark.

- *Cleanse it right:* Wash your face with slightly warm water, running it over for more than a minute. Keep dabbing warm water because it softens the face and makes it more receptive. Then wipe the water and use a cream cleanser. Gently keep going round and round all over the areas that you want to cleanse. Wipe it off with wet cotton so that your face is absolutely devoid of any dirt and grime you might have collected during the day.

+ *Wash away:* Your final step for clean skin is washing with a face wash. It removes the grime and you skin looks fresh. Take a little on your fingertips and lather, then apply all over your face, neck, and décolletage. Wash off with cold or lukewarm water depending on the weather.

When all you have and want is a pot of cream

A lot of my patients come to me with a list of concerns, and some want me to wave a magic wand! They tell me they hate to eat pills and have no patience for 10 creams...so they give me a list of what they are willing to NOT do as well.

If you are that type, let me first THANK YOU for even picking my book. And now, here's how I am going to make it all so easy for you.

Get your skin type right and then pick that one cream or lotion that suits your skin type well. So if you have oily skin, pick a lotion; if you have dry skin or mature skin, pick a pot of cream. Whatever brand it may be—it can be from La Prairie to Pond's cold cream, whatever your pocket fancies—just pick one cream.

As I have already told you, there are three things you have to do in your skincare regime—cleansing, moisturizing, and protection. Here's what you can do with one pot or bottle of potion

Remove make up: Apply the eye and lip make up, leave it on for a minute, take a warm wet cotton, and wipe it off gently. Then wipe the rest of your face and neck. No matter how much the make up, it will loosen and come off.

Exfoliate: Mix a spoonful of sugar into the lotion and apply it on your face. This acts as a gentle scrub and removes all the top dead skin cells.

You will, of course, need a face wash to wash away the residue.

As a face mask: After you have washed your face, if your skin feels dehydrated, apply a slightly thicker layer of the same cream as a face mask. Take a muslin cloth, soak it wet, and apply it over your face for 5 to 10 minutes. Rinse it off and wipe the residue. This soaks the cream really well into your skin, making it feel plump and hydrated. By doing this, your cream will behave almost like an anti-ageing cream.

As a sunscreen: Mix the cream with your make up foundation or calamine lotion and apply it on top. This will act as your sunscreen. The titanium dioxide, a sun block, is what makes these creams opaque. So that itself provides you sunscreen of about 15 SPF. This is better than anything.

As a night cream: Put some lemon juice into the cream if you need skin lightening/pore reduction and apply it thoroughly. You can also mix a few drops of essential oils like lavender if you need more hydration and have a mature skin. Put chamomile if you need calming.

Hydrant: On the days when you feel not so dry but dehydrated, wet you face slightly and apply the cream on damp skin. That acts as a moisture sealant, keeping moisture intact on the days you feel dehydrated.

Eye and lip care: Make sure you apply cream as a thick layer under your eyes and over your lips when you go to bed, so that in the morning, these areas look nice and plump.

So there you go, with just one cream, you can pretty much achieve everything you want to.

CHAPTER 11

AGEING GRACEFULLY

ONE OF MY PATIENTS once walked in with her kids, a girl aged 6 and a boy aged 1. After my session with her ended, she said her daughter had some cosmetic skin concerns too! The little girl told me that her skin felt rough while her brother's was softer and she, in her words, 'No like it'. As we age, we desire to have the skin of a baby's—chubby, plump, and soft and bouncy, so that when you pinch it, it bounces right back.

All of us see and notice what happens to the skin on top. There are enough anti-ageing products on the counter and advertisements to highlight them and educate you on signs of skin ageing. Here's a quick recap:

- ❖ Dryness that needs hydration
- ❖ Dullness that needs illuminating essence
- ❖ Dark spots and pigmentation that needs diminishing
- ❖ Wrinkles that needs to be smoothened
- ❖ Sagging skin that needs a lift

If you thought all these changes on the skin are because of ageing alone, you're mistaken.

While we grow into beautiful adults, our bone structure gets more defined, the fats go leaner, and the face gets more contoured. All this happens with the skin still glowing with youth. We love that part of ageing or 'coming of age' as we like to call it. By the time we hit 25, the tired look under the eyes, the dry skin, and may be the hollow pockets under the eyes start to bother us. A lot of people come to me at this age just saying, 'Doc I just look tired all the time, even though I sleep well and do all things right by the book.' This is when you know you are turning towards the wrong side of skin ageing. The first sign that your skin has started ageing is that it looks dehydrated. There is pigmentation, may be just a difference of tone on the face, and a few dark patches by the side of your eyes, dryness, and the pores look larger. The fine lines and creases start to show. Your skin looks dull.

Gradually you see fine lines and collagen and elastin begins to ease from the tight youthful mesh. You move to the 40s and see shadows on the cheek—the area in front of the ear—prominent laugh lines, crow's feet, frown lines, and down turned corner of the mouth with a permanent stressed out and sad expression.

If you indulge in rapid weight loss and excessive cardio, then you can even get a 'Runner's Face' i.e. gaunt, bony, and sucked out. Your body might look lean but the face does not match up, and you people asking you if you are feeling well or not, especially in India.

In your 50s, you see hollows along the temples and under eyes, cheeks sag down, and the face tends to divide into sections, with bulges over the laugh lines and jowls. Pigmentation could be a part of all of this at any age.

What you need to understand is that all that you see on your face is not what happens on the skin surface alone. So the beauty solutions may need to go beyond just application of the product on the skin alone. A lot of the symptoms are the result of what happens beneath.

We, however, know that the first sign of ageing is dryness and dullness due to the changes in the skin itself. The skin cells start to lose moisture. The ceramides that protect your epidermis also start to become less effective, leaving your skin vulnerable to outside irritants. Dead cells on top do not slough off easily and the clumped melanin stays on with it, making you look dull and darker. All of this is further aggravated through sun exposure.

Your skin defence 1

- ✦ Sunscreen
- ✦ Exfoliator
- ✦ Moisturizer
- ✦ Night cream with collagen boosters
- ✦ Omega-3 supplements
- ✦ Beauty nap (mid-day, 20 minutes)
- ✦ Good night's sleep, workouts, and balanced diet

At your skin doctor's

- ✦ Regular hydrating Medi-Facials
- ✦ Superficial peels
- ✦ Radio frequency
- ✦ Mesotherapy with non-cross linked hyaluronic acid

The second sign of ageing is change in skin tone or even pigmentation. You will also start to notice patchy skin which may be just due to the accumulation of dead cells on the top layer and the melanin clumped with it. As you age, your skin's capacity to naturally peel off the dead layer is impaired and brown spots occur due to clumping together of excessive melanin at one spot spurred by the UV rays and hormones.

Your skin defence 2

- Avoid sun between 10 am to 4 pm
- Follow all the points mentioned in the defence 1 list
- Skin lightening cream at night
- Vitamin C serum under the sunscreen
- Antioxidant oral supplement

At your skin doctor's

- Peels
- Q switched NdYag lasers
- Mesotherapy with vitamin C and other antioxidants

The third sign of ageing is thinning skin and wrinkles. As your skin ages, the collagen and elastin regenerate less and the structure gets damaged. The skin starts to thin and lines appear on various areas of your face starting with under eyes, around the eyes, around the mouth, and forehead. Prolonged and excessive exposure to harsh sun could lead to leathery thickness of the skin, what we call Solar Elastosis.

Your skin defence 3

- ❖ All on list 1
- ❖ Collagen boosting night creams
- ❖ Amino acid and essential fatty acid supplements

At your skin doctor's

- ❖ Radio frequency
- ❖ Collagen stimulating lasers
- ❖ Medium depth peels
- ❖ Micro needling
- ❖ Botox
- ❖ Platelet rich plasma

The fourth sign of ageing is facial sagging. This is where all the structures of the face come into the picture. Your features actually start to droop. The nose tip falls, the jaw and the mouth sag, and so do the eye and your brow.

After all the gyan I have given you in this section, you must know that each one of us ages differently, the reason being:

- ❖ Genes
- ❖ Lifestyle and Environment
- ❖ Attitude
- ❖ Bone structure of your face—this resorbs as you age too

If during your youthful days, you had high cheek bones, a well-defined jaw line, and arched eye brows, you will age beautifully. If on the other hand you are not so blessed with a defined bone frame and have a round face, you have to be prepared. As you grow old, you will notice your face collapsing much faster. It will bulk up at the lower part, leading to jowls and lax under the chin and neck areas. Get some fillers placed strategically just above the bone and all glory would be restored. This is where your doctor's aesthetic sense, i.e. the art with the science, counts.

Your skin defence 4

- All from list 1 and 3
- Workouts and weight training
- Vitamin D3 and calcium supplements

At your skin doctor's

FILLERS

Fillers, I tell you, are the true gift medical science gave aesthetics. They are my all-time favourite tools. The results are instant—like a blow dry for the hair—and last up to a year. I always tell my actor patients that fillers are like a theatre performance—you get to know the audience's reaction instantly and it's a great kick to the artist. It is so beautiful to see faces transform right in front of you, unlike lasers and other treatments where we work long sessions and repeatedly many a times and the results are like a movie that releases months later.

Contributing structures under the skin

Ageing and your facial muscles. The other component that contributes to your beauty are the facial muscles.

Unlike the rest of the body, they are attached to the skin above and not the bone below. So each time they contract to make an expression, they drag the skin along which leads to the formation of expression lines. Botox can be your saviour here. This does not mean lessening your facial expressions. It's about selectively relaxing the muscles to an extent that the unwanted negative and depressing expression lines are removed.

This picture shows the negative and positive expressions.

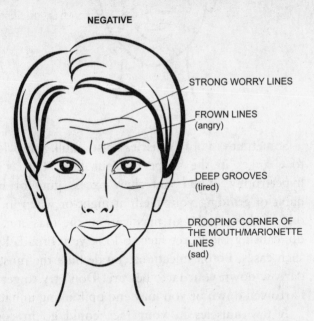

NEGATIVE

STRONG WORRY LINES

FROWN LINES
(angry)

DEEP GROOVES
(tired)

DROOPING CORNER OF
THE MOUTH/MARIONETTE
LINES
(sad)

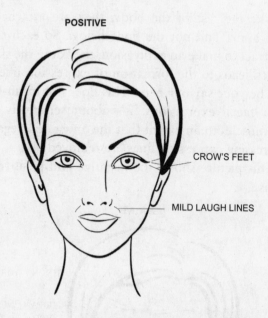

POSITIVE

CROW'S FEET

MILD LAUGH LINES

Sometimes your muscles also bulk up, leading to changes in the shape of your face. This is called hypertrophy. When you chew excess gum or have a habit of grinding your teeth at night or when in stress, one of the muscles of mastication, the masseter, bulks up, causing the lower face to look very broad. Even in such cases, Botox injections can de-bulk the muscles to narrow down your face. Beware! Don't try to get it too narrowed down or you may end up looking unnatural.

A few muscles in your face could go in constant contraction, like the depressor at the corners of your mouth. This makes you look sad all the time with a down turned mouth. Minute shots of Botox into that muscle is all it takes to put the joy back in your smile. Other features like the brow shape and the dipping tip of

FACIAL MUSCLES

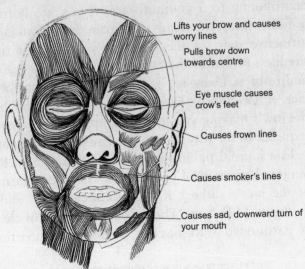

Lifts your brow and causes worry lines

Pulls brow down towards centre

Eye muscle causes crow's feet

Causes frown lines

Causes smoker's lines

Causes sad, downward turn of your mouth

your nose can all be beautified with Botox. Also, Botox applied to the Platysma muscle on the jaw line helps you stop tugging your face down. This treatment is popularly called Nefertiti treatment.

THE IDEAL NOSE

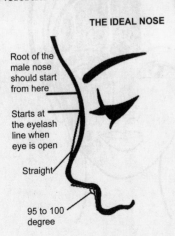

Root of the male nose should start from here

Starts at the eyelash line when eye is open

Straight

95 to 100 degree

Facial fat pockets are another important component contributing to a youthful face. If you are born with a fuller face, you tend to remain fresh looking and attractive most of the times. If not, the first sign of tiredness sets in as the fat pocket under your eye shifts and resorbs. Likewise, fat in the other sections of your face either resorbs like the cheeks or descend like in the jowls making you look less attractive. They have a sequence in the way they show change while you age.

In a journal published by the Department of Plastic Surgery, University of Texas, titled 'The fat compartments of the face', authors Rod J. Rohrich, M.D. and Joel E. Pessa, M.D. say, 'The subcutaneous fat of the face is partitioned into discrete anatomic compartments.

THE SUBCUTANEOUS FAT COMPARTMENTS OF THE FACE

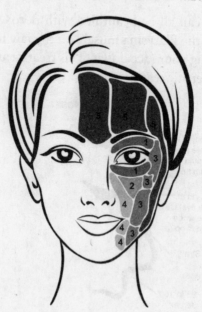

Facial ageing is, in part, characterized by how these compartments change with age.' The numbers in this picture indicate the order in which these fat pockets are affected as you age.

Your beauty defence

- Do not lose weight drastically
- Consume at least 2 spoons of oil/ghee per day
- Take essential fatty oil supplements

At your skin doctor's

- Fillers to add what is lost
- Lipo dissolve to dissolve what has bulged up and decended

The ageing timeline

Age 25–30: Visible ageing begins when the skin cell renewal starts to slow down.

Age 30–35: Expression lines become more prominent as collagen and elastin start to break down.

Age 35–40: Static lines begin to appear. Skin starts to thin. Skin becomes noticeably more dry. Shift of facial fats become noticeable.

Age 40 onwards: The change may suddenly be visible, especially with Indian skin types. If you are petite with a good bone structure and stable body weight, you would have enjoyed a blessed skin up until now, and at 40 it all seems to suddenly give up—skin, face, and body!

Age 50 onwards: Facial muscles sag along with the other structures like fat. Bone framework and teeth support is compromised and skin appears fragile.

Age Erase in Your Teens

When you hit your teens, it is most likely that your seesawing hormones start playing havoc with your skin. While you cannot avoid little zits and breakouts once in a while as your body adjusts itself, a good skincare regime can see you through the toughest skin phase of your life.

As a teenager, your skincare regime is different from your mom's. It's definitely much simpler, and you do not need a cupboard full of beauty potions. Your skincare routine should be about proper cleansing and protecting your skin's natural oil and moisture balance.

It is a good idea to invest in a good cleanser and moisturizer meant for younger skin. Avoid using creams meant for your mother, as they are formulated to handle older skin, which is very different from a young person's skin.

Here's what you need

- Make sure you wash your hands with a hand wash soap each time before you wash your face.
- Do not keep touching your skin.
- Washing your face 3 times a day is a must.
- Do not pinch or poke your acne.
- Make sunscreen your best friend.

❖ Whiteheads and blackheads are blocked oil glands, so do not try to scratch them. Get professional help instead.

❖ Dandruff can cause trouble on your face, back, and shoulder skin.

❖ Acne can be bad in the long-term and needs to be addressed right away.

❖ Laser hair reduction is a safe procedure and it takes about a year to get good results, so if you are planning to move towns to study, plan it right.

❖ Make up will not harm your skin. What harms is not removing it.

❖ A well-balanced diet is absolutely essential.

Those worrisome skin woes

Excessive oiliness: As your hormonal levels rise and body changes, so does your skin. Suddenly the pores open up, and there is an excessive production of sebum, and thus your skin looks shiny and sticky at all times. Your first reaction will be to use a soap every time to wash off the oiliness. But do not over wash your skin so much so that it dries up the skin. This can actually have an adverse reaction with your glands going on an overdrive to maintain the balance. Instead, use a face wash meant for oily skin, and use a facial mist and a muslin cloth to wipe away excess oil in between cleansing without stripping your skin. Also, use a water-based moisturizer or a light skin lotion.

Acne: As you start on your menstrual cycle, you will notice that your skin breaks out into acne. For some it is an occasional event while for others it can be a chronic condition. Acne can present itself as whiteheads, blackheads, or pus filled pimples. It usually develops in the central area of the cheeks and on the forehead, and it's almost universally caused by a hormone imbalance or a hypersensitivity to the robust hormonal activity going on the body during this time. Stress can also aggravate this condition. Treatments with benzoyl peroxide or salicylic acid works.

HOME CARE FOR ACNE

- ❖ *Yeast, lemon juice and water:* Make a paste and apply on the spot. Leave for ten minutes and wash off
- ❖ *Holy basil toner*: Boil tulsi or basil in water, reduce, and leave it to cool. Use this after washing your face to ward off oiliness and impending acne
- ❖ Sandal wood paste
- ❖ Wash your hair daily

Sweating: Be it on the palms of your hands and soles of your feet, under your arms, in your scalp, or anywhere on your body, if you often find yourself drenched in perspiration, you're not alone. Blame your seesawing changes inside.

- ❖ Carry tissues and wet wipes.
- ❖ Some aluminium compounds act by blocking sweat when applied, like All Dry.
- ❖ If the sweating is excessive and bothering you, try Botox. It is a medically approved treatment.

Age Erase in Your 20s

After the terrible teens, when your skin just goes topsy-turvy, it is in your 20s that you see your skin settling down and glowing with natural youthfulness. Don't take that glow and shine for granted. Your carefree lifestyle, lack of sleep, endless partying, alcohol, smoke, and often neglect of the skin can give rise to skin issues and start the ageing process faster than you may like.

The three best things that you can do to keep this natural glow and suppleness for longer are:

- Eat a balanced diet at the right times
- Get enough sleep, and **do not** smoke
- Skin doesn't mind an occasional glass of drink
- Get into a skin routine
- If you have acne, go get medical help

Most young women in their early 20s do not really think about what all-night parties and roaming in the sun without sunscreen can do to their skin. The first signs of ageing you start noticing as you hit your 25th year is dryness, under eye hollowness, and uneven skin tone.

In your 20s your main skin goal should be to preserve and protect. Regular skin cleansing and protection should be your key beauty ritual.

Your 4-step regimen:

Step 1: Use a gentle foaming cleanser that will remove make up and excess oil but won't dry out your skin. Once a week you can try a mild scrub to remove tanning and dull skin.

Step 2: For daytime, use a light moisturizer that contains sunscreen with UVA and UVB protection. Or just pick up a broad spectrum sunscreen. If you suffer from acne, then do some spot treatments with salicylic acid.

Look for hydrating creams with some skin brightening optical illusion properties in them that brightens your skin immediately and doubles up as make up.

Step 3: If you have irregular sleep cycles and spend lot of nights staying up, then add an antioxidant like vitamin C and Omega fatty acids to your diet as well as your skincare regime. You can look for creams with pomegranate, grape seed extracts, *amla* or Indian gooseberry, or vitamin C, and Co Q 10. You can pick a serum to use under your sunscreen or make up. Try some face packs on your day off to pep up your skin and give it that little extra it needs.

Step 4: At night, after washing your face, you can apply a hydrating mask or a layer of your cream or moisturizer. Clean off before you hit the bed.

Hair Care

In your 20s your hair might look and feel great, but this is also the time when most of us put it through the test. Partying hard means more styling products, harsh chemical treatments whether colouring, perming or straightening, and not to forget sun damage. You must use a gentle shampoo to wash your hair every day, especially during summer days, and especially if you use styling products. Do not forget to use your conditioner. If you know you are going to be out in the sun, then use a sun protection serum. Also before using heat styling tools, coat your hair with some heat protecting hair sprays to avoid cuticle damage. Make sure you are massaging your hair and scalp at least twice a week with oil to keep them healthy.

FEW HAIR FACTS

- Blow drying is any day better than ironing. Direct heat on the hair damages it the most.
- Let the wind from the blow dryer hit your hair along the hair cuticle and not against them. This will lift the cuticles and make your hair strands rough and brittle.
- Use a heat protectant before you blow dry.
- Never iron wet or damp hair.
- Oil not only scalp but all along the hair strand. It is actually the later part of your hair length that needs oil the most.
- What you eat tells on your hair as well.
- Hormones and your nutrition status affect the quality of hair.
- Sugar in your diet makes hair brittle.
- Do not use tight hair accessories.
- Don't comb wet hair.
- Using hair mousse as a volumizer is not a good idea.
- Any form of styling heat on mousse is a BIG NO.

For Men

I think men in their 20s are least bothered about how they look or feel. Yes, they might spend some time on shaving and styling their hair, but they really do not think they need any skincare other than their aftershave lotion. Well, boys out there, you guys are so wrong. You are more prone to acne, open pores, and oily skin than girls, so you need to keep your face clean. The right face wash that has salysilic acid or benzoyl peroxide or tea tree oil and which foams well is essential, especially as soon as you get back from the outdoors. When you are going out, please do not forget your sunscreen. One of the most common concerns men come to my clinic with is pigmentation on the sides of their forehead and temples! Sun care is very important for men too. Do not keep rubbing the sweat off your forehead. Friction can cause skin pigmentation.

Beard conditioner

Yes, even if you think you don't need it, we women think you do! If you are not clean shaved, you may be responsible for the skin rash that your daughter or wife may have, so please use beard softeners or simply use a hair conditioner. Leave it on for 5 minutes and rinse it off. Your stubble will not be so abrasive after this procedure.

At your skin doctor's

If you have an acne prone skin, then first go for a panel of blood investigations and ultrasound of your pelvis to rule out any internal causes. Then come peels and extractions and light therapy for acne, along with necessary medication. Also do not forget to try some hydrating treatments as acne medication can over dry your skin like hydra facials.

If you have had acne in your teens and have remnant scars, then go for peels or lasers depending on the colour and type of scar. You can then go for a pigment laser or a collagen stimulating laser/radio frequency/micro needling .

If you are blessed with great skin, then maintain it with occasional exfoliating treatments like peels and then start with the hair reduction lasers, right skincare routine. Fillers may be for facial enhancement like cheek bone, chin enhancement, lip enhancement. Botox for brow, jaw line shaping etc. Yes, at times the negative expression lines can start soon and then it is best to treat them before they turn into passive lines and need more work.

People prone to more sun exposure should know that for others ageing changes start in their early 20s, but for them it starts a bit sooner. So you can start with skin pigment lasers and collagen stimulating lasers and radio frequencies.

It's never too early to start taking care. Start prevention, start your journey towards graceful ageing, but make sure you go to the right place for help.

Age Erase in Your 30s

So you have hit the big 3 'oh's! You have a good career, a good set of friends, and more stability in life than before. More importantly, you are done with student life and feel all grown up! But this is the time when you are also starting to worry just a bit when you look at the mirror. Maybe, you spot a hint of fine line or extra pigment. Yes, it is time to visit your doctor.

As you progress in your 30s, some of the signs of photo-ageing start to show up. Especially, as you cross your

35th year, you will notice more pigmentation and dull skin issues. But if you have been religiously following a good skincare routine in your younger years, the impact might be less.

Anti-ageing treatment does not mean that you address it after you see the first wrinkle. Take the preventive care approach. If you take care now, then your skin will thank you much later. Ageing for me does not mean the number of candles on your cake, but how your skin looks and feels. So before pigmentation and fine lines become a challenge, try this regime.

The most important thing is to find a right exfoliating face wash or scrub that goes well with your skin type. This illuminates your skin and keeps it soft and supple.

Your 5-step regimen:

Step 1: Continue with the regime you set up in your 20s. You may add a little more to your cleansing routine. Use the combination of make up remover and a face wash to get really clean skin. In your cleansing routine, add a gentle scrub every alternate night. You can also look for a face wash that contains some exfoliating actives like AHA. This is because your skin's natural sloughing off process starts to slow down now.

Step 2: Take special care of the under eye area and lips. Use a lightening, capillary stabilizing cream like Vit K, blood pigment clearing lotion like Arnica under-eye gel or cream every night. Use a concealer with a good moisturizer during the day. Sunscreen is important here too. For eye and lip care refer to the earlier chapter. Use beeswax-based lip butter with an SPF to keep them soft.

EARLY OR MILD CHANGES

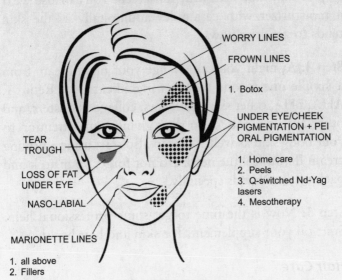

WORRY LINES

FROWN LINES

1. Botox

UNDER EYE/CHEEK
PIGMENTATION + PEI
ORAL PIGMENTATION

1. Home care
2. Peels
3. Q-switched Nd-Yag lasers
4. Mesotherapy

TEAR TROUGH

LOSS OF FAT UNDER EYE

NASO-LABIAL

MARIONETTE LINES

1. all above
2. Fillers

MODERATE AGEING CHANGES

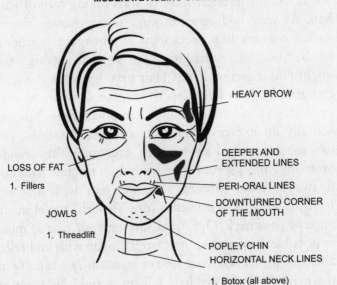

HEAVY BROW

DEEPER AND EXTENDED LINES

PERI-ORAL LINES

DOWNTURNED CORNER OF THE MOUTH

LOSS OF FAT

1. Fillers

JOWLS

1. Threadlift

POPLEY CHIN

HORIZONTAL NECK LINES

1. Botox (all above)

Step 3: Continue with your sunscreen. You can also wear a moisturizer with ceramides additionally as the skin tends to get drier now.

Step 4: At night you can change your night cream from a simple one to one that has ingredients like Retin A, AHA, BHA, other skin lighteners, collagen boosters, and other anti oxidants. Also start giving some attention to your body skin as well. You can also start using a firming cream if you feel the need. Do not forget your neck and back of your hands specially.

Step 5: Now is the time to get some professional help. Start on your supplements for skin and hair health.

Hair Care

30s is when you really have to start taking care of your hair. As your body goes through some changes due to varied reasons like pregnancy or changing hormonal levels, your hair starts to show signs of ageing. You might find it getting frizzy. Hair gets dry while the scalp can get oily. Hair fall starts to become an issue. So keep up with your oil massage and shampoo regime. You can actually do it every alternate day. Post shampoo, you can use a protein hair mask to strengthen the strands. Start applying a serum after washing it to tame frizz and flyaways. Avoid rubbing your wet hair with a towel. Instead, wrap it in a muslin (not Turkish) towel at the nape of your neck. Opt for air-drying your hair as much as possible. Protect your hair from the sun with umbrellas and sun protection hair sprays now easily available in the market. If you see hair fall, this could be a sign of hormonal imbalance. Common at this age are polycystic ovaries or iron deficiency leading to anaemia.

> **WHY SELF-READING MEDICAL REPORTS IS A BIG NO-NO!**
>
> A lots of us tend to self-read our blood reports, see that our numbers are within the normal range, and skip going back to the doctor. That's a big mistake! The normal ranges could be anywhere between 4 to 400, but what you need for optimum health will be either somewhere in-between, some hormones in the upper one-third, and some others in the lower third of the range. For example, you look at your haemoglobin percentage and feel happy when it's in range. If it is borderline but within range, it is entirely possible that you will still feel all the symptoms of anaemia, be it tiredness or dark circles or hair fall.

PROTEIN INFUSION FOR YOUR HAIR

Apply egg on your head. Or whisk an egg with some yogurt and apply the mask over your hair and scalp. Leave it on for a while. Shampoo and condition as usual. If you can't stand the smell, then add a few drops of lavender essential oil. It has a calming effect on irritated scalp.

For Men

Continue with your cleansing, moisturizing, and suncare routine. However, now is a good time to use a moisturizer with some vitamins and antioxidants to fight the skin ageing process. You can also go for professional facials to hydrate your skin, and maybe to fight that tan.

At your skin doctor's

- ❖ Gentle acid peels.
- ❖ Botox for frown lines and few under eye lines.
- ❖ Fillers mostly under eyes or on your lips to give you a pout or to give it better definition.
- ❖ PRP(Platelet Rich Plasma) which is your own plasma enriched with platelets and growth factors re-injected with micro-needles that stimulate collagen and hydrate your skin. Peps up the skin that might have just about begun to slow down.
- ❖ Skin tightening and lightening lasers.
- ❖ Radio frequency along with micro needling which gives a deeper stimulation so aids good collagen stimulation. Also helps acne scars if you have been suffering from them all this while. You get both skin tightening and texture improvement from this treatment and if need be, lessen some fat from the cheek area along with fat dissolving injections.

VAMPIRE THERAPY, ANYONE?

Vampire Therapy, also called PRP (Plasma Rich Platelet) Therapy is recommended for anyone who prefers a more natural approach to anti-ageing or scar revision treatments. This treatment involves taking the patient's blood and separating the blood components. We at Ra Skin 'n' Aesthetics use an FDA-approved Swiss patented technology gel which enriches the platelets with growth factor, which on injection into the skin cause skin rejuvenation and tissue regeneration, leading to improved skin vitality, and a smoother, hydrated, more elastic skin with a youthful appearance by means of

---

- ❖ Biostimulation of stem cells by growth factors from your own plasma
- ❖ Revitalizing and regenerating dermis cells
- ❖ Supporting new collagen formation
- ❖ Smoothening out wrinkles and folds
- ❖ Increasing density and luminosity of your skin with reduction of wrinkles and fine lines and fading of dark circles

It is not only great for skin rejuvenation, it works wonders in the most natural way for hair thinning and hair fall too. Most popular among balding men or men with a definite history of balding in the family, this treatment should be undertaken when they start to notice increase in hair fall. You'll be surprised that balding is a bigger issue than any skin concern in my male patients! It also works great on women who have hair thinning problems post pregnancy or stressful times or post menopause. Even a couple of sittings done a month apart makes a great difference in the thickness and health of existing hair and growth of new hair.

Prevention with Botox. Is it possible?

YES, it is absolutely possible. What is facial ageing? As I said earlier, the change in the structures from the skin down to the bone, muscle, and gravity plays a major role. There are by and large two sets of muscles: one set that pulls everything up or in one direction and another set that antagonises or pulls everything in the other direction. Likewise on the face too there are muscles that pull your brow, the corner of your eye, the corner of your mouth, and the entire lower part of your face down towards the neck called platysma. If I ease these with Botox, the other set that pulls them up gains more strength. So voila! You can slow down the signs of ageing but make sure you go to an expert doctor with a good aesthetic practice.

Age Erase in Your 40s

In your 40s, you have officially matured, and now you are seriously stressed out. The same lifestyle may feel a bit more taxing; the same food seems to turn into instant fat. You have regulated your lifestyle, yet you look pale and tired. Your skin is sagging and you are seriously packing on weight, especially around your belly. Your face is now showing your expression lines and the lines around your brows and eyes do not disappear, not matter how much you try. Your skin feels dry and looks thin.

Okay, so before you push the panic button, it's time you start a routine for your skin at home with the right products, preferably after consulting your doctor. If you have already done that, revisit the same doctor for a review. What you used all this while may not be enough and may not even be right for your skin concerns now. You need to now add extra moisture and collagen building actives into your skin to give it all the help you can. Start taking supplements that help your skin. Do not cut all oils from your diet as they help in keeping the skin lubricated.

ADVANCED AGEING CHANGES

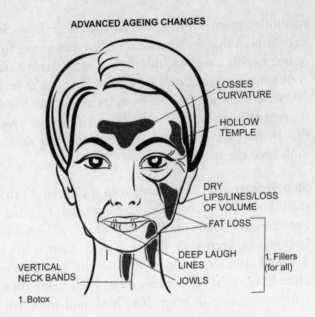

LOSSES CURVATURE

HOLLOW TEMPLE

DRY LIPS/LINES/LOSS OF VOLUME

FAT LOSS

DEEP LAUGH LINES

1. Fillers (for all)

VERTICAL NECK BANDS

JOWLS

1. Botox

Your 4-Step Regime:

Step 1: Your cleansing routine now needs to get more gentle and one that adds moisture to your skin. If your skin feels very dry, you can shift from gel face wash to creamy face wash that will not strip away the natural oils from your skin. Try a 5-minute quick massage with oil or cream before using a face wash. This not only provides moisture but also stimulates your skin, reducing puffiness. Refer to the chapter on massage to get your strokes right.

Step 2: Your day care should have a serum with anti-oxidants to fight free radicals and help reverse some of the damage you have already done. It can also have some anti-inflammatory properties to soothe dryness. Studies have shown that inflammation is the key cause to most of our health issues including skin acne, ageing etc. Use your sunscreen religiously. Pick one that has at least SPF 30. Whether you have dark circles or not, do not forget to use an under eye cream under and over your eyes since this is the part that gives up your age and makes you look tired the most.

Step 3: Start your night care with a cleansing ritual and then your 5-minute face massage and relaxing neck exercises like head rotation, and while your head is flung backwards, keep your mouth closed. That way you get a stretch and extra blood rush to the area below your chin. Your night time cream should be thicker than what you were using in your 30s. It should primarily have some skin lightening properties to fight the dullness that the skin tends to settle with. You can use creams with peptides, retinol, liquorice, Kojic acid, and hyaluronic acid.

Step 4: It's time to visit your skin doctor. If you want to keep it basic, then start with good vitamin and antioxidant infusion facials every 15 days. Go for a collagen stimulating laser once a month for around 6 sittings to start with. You can also opt for sessions of radio frequency.

If you are a little more open to injections, then mesotherapy is a very beneficial treatment to go for.

If you seriously want to look your best now, you can try shots of Botox and fillers. This really does the magic. Trust me, a drop of filler under your eyes and cheeks can brighten your whole face and your mood too.

Also kick start your physical workout—try some weight training or yoga. This will keep your muscles toned, bones strong, and also up your happy hormones.

Hair Care

The biggest worry is that hair starts to thin, and grey strands become noticeable. You can blame it on the reduced oestrogen levels, and increased Dihydrotestosteron (DHT) in some cases which can really constrict your roots. Also do not forget to check your thyroid function at this stage. This means thinner strands and restricted growth. You can colour your hair with ammonia-free colours as they are gentler on the strands. Look for natural plant colours since they will preserve your hair in the long run. You may have to do those touch ups for the rest of your life. A good idea is to touch up just the crown, partition line, and the entire hair only once in 6 months. Go for regular hair spa treatments. Specific hair supplements with vitamins like biotine specially improve hair health. Shift to a gentler shampoo and conditioner—preferably hydrating and colour protecting variants.

At your skin doctor's

+ Continue with gentle acid peels and Medi-Facials.
+ Botox can now be directed to those vertical bands on the neck, and the horizontal lines along your upper face. I do not believe in knocking off all the forehead lines or worry lines which can be done by working on a muscle called frontalis. This is the only muscle that lifts your brow up, so a few lines can make you look natural. You'd rather preserve

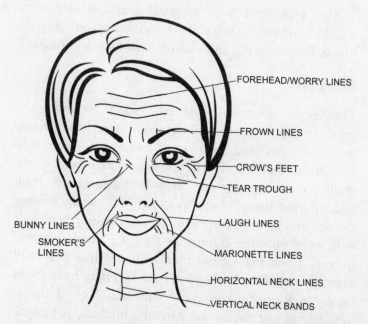

FOREHEAD/WORRY LINES

FROWN LINES

CROW'S FEET

TEAR TROUGH

BUNNY LINES

SMOKER'S LINES

LAUGH LINES

MARIONETTE LINES

HORIZONTAL NECK LINES

VERTICAL NECK BANDS

the brow lifting function. However, feel free to knock off those vertical frown lines between your brow. Working on the lateral third of your eyebrow can give a good lift and make your eyes look open and wide.

❖ Fillers: This does the magic when used on the cheek to give a super face lift. Make sure it is placed right and just enough on the deeper lines like the laugh lines and corners of your mouth. A little filler on the chin at this age gives a lot of lift to the lower face.

❖ Mesotherapy: With a non-crosslinked hyaluronic acid, it will give a very good deep hydration along with collagen stimulation. It really plumps your skin to make it look youthful.

- Skin tightening and lightening lasers.
- Radio frequency.
- Start extending peels and lasers on to your décolletage and back of your hands.

Also at my clinic, we do alternating mesotherapy with hair stimulating formulations and platelet rich plasma that gives amazing results.

Age Erase in Your 50s

This, as I see it, is the most beautiful stage of anyone's life. I often look at my patients in this age group with envy. They have such a glow on their faces radiating from within, having achieved so much on personal and professional fronts, having understood life and made peace with it all. Ladies, by this time you are done with the menopause issues as well. So what if there are a few lines and pigmentation problem and tissue descent? What is medical science for? What is the skin doctor for? I remember my granny telling me, 'What are you doctors for if I have to stop myself from consuming sugar in all forms just to keep my diabetes under control.' She happily ate what she fancied and blamed the doctor each time. So my lovely readers, let's do some simple stuff. Now that you have taken care of the whole world, this is your time.

If you have been diligent about your skincare from the beginning, then you are lucky because I am sure your skin ageing will be much less apparent. However,

I suggest that you invest in products that offer higher treatment actives.

Your 4-Step regimen:

Step 1: Use a cream cleanser not just to wash your face but also your hands and neck. It will fight the crepey texture that may bother you. Massage is a great friend for the face and the body. You can do it pre-bath and post bath with a nice body oil. Choose light oils like coconut or may be jojoba, avocado, or macadamia nut oil if you can get any one of these. If you are going for oiling after taking a bath, then apply it on damp skin so it preserves hydration and gives you moisture. The skin may start to get itchy at this age due to lack of oestrogen in women and because of skin thinning out.

Step 2: All your day care products should have some sort of SPF. You can apply a thin layer of day cream before applying the sunscreen. If you use make up, you can opt for liquid foundation that is not too powdery or with matte finish. Eye and lip care is a must.

Step 3: Rich, creamy moisturizer with anti-ageing properties should be your best friend. Before applying a cream, apply a serum with de-pigmentation and anti-ageing properties. After it soaks into the skin, apply your peptide and ceramide, oil-enriched night cream. Do not forget your neck and hands as well.

Step 4: You can try out skin tightening laser treatments and some fillers as well. All the treatments at 40 can continue now or started at this stage as well.

Yoga is the way to go, especially anti-gravity positions. Also a bit of weight training will keep your bones and joints intact.

At your skin doctor's

- Go for stronger acid peels. With our Indian skin type, we may not be good with deep strong peels, but we do well with leave-on peels which keep working and sloughing off top layers of the skin over a week, like some Retin A peels, popularly known as yellow peels, or Kojic acid peels that also work well on pigmentation. Your doctor applies it and sends you home to keep it on for over 5 to 6 hours or at times even overnight.

- By this age, I suggest my patients to not do away with all their facial lines. Forehead worry lines, also the lines by the side of your eyes, actually make your smile look even more beautiful and one would look unnatural with no lines at all at 50 and above. However, a few eaed muscles gives you a very relaxed look. The key is to keep it natural.

- Fillers: If you have not tried fillers yet, this is the time. You could achieve a very natural and a no-down time face lift which takes just an hour of your time! Everyone will notice and no one will be able to tell. But let me warn you, this will work only if an expert doctor does this. Look at yourself in the mirror—the tissue or volume loss is all over, bit by bit from the sides of your forehead, between your brows, temples, cheeks in the front, and by the side of your ears. All the tissue seems to collect and move down to the front of your face next to the nose and mouth and the jowls. Therefore, it needs to be volumed as well. Fillers are a great tool and you'll see a fresh, youthful face right after the procedure.

❖ Extend all procedures to the hands, neck and décolletage, including fillers.
❖ Skin tightening and lightening lasers.
❖ Radio frequency.

Age Erase in Your 60s and Beyond

You could now belong to one of these four categories:

1. You have been working on your face for some years now with your aesthetic doctors.
2. Followed good home care with no intervention at all.
3. Just didn't bother but had a healthy skin lifestyle.
4. Did nothing towards skin and hair health. Instead you sun bathed, surfed, ate and drank mindlessly.

Category 1

I applaud you. You will now be getting all the compliments while you are out with your contemporaries. I knew of a set of identical twins out of whom one was injected, layered, got great home care for 5 years of her life, and then stopped all invasive treatments, and the other who was not really intervened with at all. 10 years later, a picture of theirs showed that the one who was worked on for 5 years looked way more beautiful and youthful than the other. So if you are one of those who are scared what happens if you are not regular, you are still better off. So now back to your scenario...yes, you look super for your age. So keep going at it.

Your focus should now be on

Skin hydration, so use the right oils and liquids in your diet and apply thicker, more enriching cream over damp skin as fat under the skin shrinks. Your skin might be so dry that you may experience severe itching on the areas where the skin is stretched over the bone, for example your shin. Keep your bath super short and mix a spoon of oil in the last mug of water. Use oils like coconut on damp body.

At your skin doctor's

Hyaluronic acid injections just under the skin will give you instant and longer gratification along with collagen stimulation.

A. Sun protection

Apply sunscreen on top of your moisturizers and below your coloured make-up. Avoid going out in the sun between 11 am and 4 pm. Use an antioxidant below the sunscreen as free radical damage is one thing that your sunscreen can't do anything about. Once you are inside, don't forget to calm your skin with calamine mixed with a moisturizer. Also by now it is good for you to use warm water than cold water.

B. Skin colour, pigmentation

Your skin colour could be becoming darker with every passing year due to the accumulation of dead skin cells with pigments in them. In such a case, use a face wash with glycolic acid or go for regular peels at your doctor's. Refer to the pigmentation chapter for various other forms of pigmentation. The remedies remain the same, no matter what age you are. Second, the skin could be going pale. This is due to the thinning of skin, loss of fat under the skin, lack of proper blood flow etc. Get more stimulating massages done and go for warm water washes. Exercise to keep your bones and muscles strong and your skin firm.

C. SKIN SAGGING

After you cross 60, stimulating new collagen may be not as good as it was in your younger days. So if you choose to try treatments at your doctor's, you could ease your expectations from the lasers, lights, and radio frequencies. Instead, volume and structural correction will give more firmness to the skin. However, keep the Retin As and the peptides going in your night creams, with some good exfoliation.

D. KEEP UP THE STRUCTURE

If you have been in good hands, this should not be of a concern now. Maybe a bit of a filler here and there will keep it going and a few units of Botox can be applied to the muscles that keep pulling your face downwards.

Category 2

Your skin should be great in terms of sun protection, hydration, firmness, and tone since you are taking care. If you're facing any particular concern, then based on your needs, refer to the previous chapters.

But most importantly, what you may now have to look into are the procedures that I have talked about in category 1 for all the sections A, B, and C.

However, you may need a lot of work on the structural and muscle activity that may have created lines, active and passive, volume, and structural loss.

Keep up the facial structures. This is one of the most important factors at this stage. Find a good dentist as the height of your teeth are shortened as you age and so your mouth/lip puckers inward. Also there is loss of bone mineralization and so bone volume reduces. At my clinic, I work with fillers to give you a face lift effect with no down time and very harmonious and natural look.

Category 3

All of you in this category need to start with a general health assessment. Get all your nutrients and hormones right, and get in touch with a fitness consultant to get on a fitness program. Then move on to sun protection, moisturization, and a good facial cleanser. Get used to having a skincare regimen. You'll realize that it is not too bad. All it takes is 5 minutes each time. Just sheer touching and firm stroking can make you love your skin so much more and increase your beauty. Make sure all your strokes are with the flat end of your fingers and not the full palm. Use gentle yet firm upward strokes. Do not forget the neck, décolletage and limbs, or for that matter, your entire body.

Category 4

People in this category have been so high on life that they haven't had time to pay any attention to their skin or follow a particular routine as such. Your skin and hair require regimental discipline over a period of time to show a certain result and such people may not have the patience or inclination to do it. So if people in this category want to go back to what they 'could have had', they should start with skin boosters just underneath the skin which will take care of hydration, sun damage, fine wrinkles, the 'deflated' look, and a little bit of volume loss on the surface which is pretty much the most important thing you want to be addressed. The results will encourage you to follow the schedule more religiously. My dad, who is 75 now, was so careful about keeping his skin hydrated always. In fact, I've never seen him step out without moisturizing his body every single morning and has minimal sun exposure. Oh, I love his skin! In fact my daughter often tells me she wished her skin was like her grandpa's.

Special Care for Other Features

Special care for your eyes

When you age, what ages first are your eyes, or the tissues under it.

- ❖ As I mentioned previously, the skin around the eyes is very thin, thinner than the rest of your body, so it tends to wrinkle easily. Moisturize with a collagen boosting cream, one with hyaluronic acid, vitamin E, Retin A (low concentrations), and preferably all 3 together. But if that's unavailable, do not hesitate to use 2 or 3 creams and apply them one over the other or at different times, in which case Retin A is always applied only at night. Try mesotherapy with PRP or non-crosslinked hyaluronic acid; both stimulate collagen and hydrate intensely.

- Eyes have no oil glands of their own so they tend to get really dry. The wrinkles and skin sensitivity only makes matters worse. To reduce irritation, use eye cream rich in moisture and calming ingredients like calamine.

- The fine capillaries are very delicate. So if you have the habit of rubbing your eyes, apply cream in the wrong direction, or remove make up the wrong way, you risk rupturing those capillaries. The leak from those capillaries can give you dark circles.

Common eye concerns

DARK CIRCLES

Dark circles can be caused due to structural contributors like deep set eyes and therefore, the shadow of the brow casting a dark circle on the area below your eye, under eye fat regressing due to age, or the one common thing that most Indians are born with which is the tear trough—all make you look tired and cause dark circles. The structural ones are easiest to treat. All they need is a shot of filler and your eyes look instantly bright.

Another cause for dark circles can be the dark colour of the skin. This can happen due to various reasons and so the treatments are many too. Below are a few causes of dark circles:

1. Familial, i.e. someone in your family may have it too and you may have had it for as long as you remember, so to lighten this is difficult. But skin lightening creams, lasers, and peels can achieve quite a bit.
2. Dark grey due to deeper pigmentation or then deposition of blood pigment called hemosiderin that is left over from the capillary leak. Use creams with vitamin K or Arnica.
3. Large veins underneath give a blue undertone. Some fillers added in the layer between the vein and skin helps as does radio frequency that facilitates skin thickness with collagen regeneration.
4. Simple iron deficiency: Anaemia-supplements under a doctor's guidance will result in a great change.
5. Lifestyle: Though I mention this the last, this is most important.

UNDER EYE BAGS

One of my patients once told me, 'Nothing can upset me more than when I wake up with a bag under my eye, especially before my periods.' True, under eye bags can be a traumatizing experience for many. But there can be different reasons for under eye bags including various medical conditions.

- *Water retention:* When water the bulge, it becomes less prominent when you gaze up. Also, it is not restricted to the margin of the bone around the eye. This is due to your normal cycles and fluid retention before-periods, or due to more serious issues like thyroid. You will get relief by contracting and relaxing your eye muscles, sleeping with a double pillow, and reducing the after-sunset salt content in your diet.
- *Fat from under eye muscle:* This is more defined and is restricted to the bone margin. It becomes more prominent on looking up and is best removed surgically. Use filler around it to even it out. Fillers help if the fat is minimal.
- *Malar fat pad:* You see a triangle sort of island in the outer half of the under eye. This is a small pad of fat separated by attachments of the skin to the bone beneath. It may get more prominent as you age. Surgical or filler corrections are your options.

If you look at this at different stages of life, then at 30s you will start noticing dark circles and some dryness around the eye area. Fine lines too start to show. Also the under eye area starts to get hollow as the surrounding fat pocket starts to regress. This leads to sunken eyes which can make you look tired.

In your 40s, crow's feet start to get prominent. The crow's feet seems to stay there even when you are not laughing. The sunken area gets more defined, and sometimes deep lines starts to appear which divides your cheeks into two. Over the eyelids, your brow starts to droop. In your 50s, the same signs get more accentuated.

Along with this, there is loss of fat above the eye, mostly all around the eye socket. The tail of the brow droops to lie heavily on the eye.

HOW TO GET BRIGHT BEAUTIFUL EYES:

Creams to be applied under the eye.

- **Moisturizer:** to rehydrate and plump the thin dry skin.
- **Calming agents:** to reduce the redness and inflammation
- **Arnica or vitamin K:** to avoid capillary breakage and leaks by stablizing the capillaries and easing off the blood components that may be contributing to the dark skin.
- **Skin lightening substances** like Kojic Acid, turmeric extract, or very mild Hydroquinone.
- **Anti-oxidants:** Vitamin C will protect and lighten the area
- Vitamin E will keep the skin soft and supple.

The cream should be soft, creamy, and smooth in texture. Always note how it feels on your skin when you apply the cream. Avoid something that feels too sticky or heavy. Try a fragrance-free product and one that has fewer preservatives. Pick creams that have lesser number of ingredients so that the chances of irritation are reduced. Always use gentle strokes from outside inwards on the lower eyelid and inside outwards on the upper eyelid area with the ball of your finger.

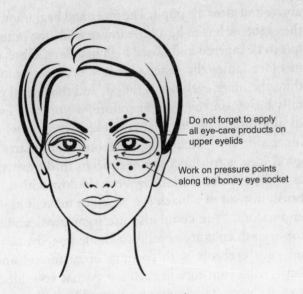

Do not forget to apply all eye-care products on upper eyelids

Work on pressure points along the boney eye socket

When you put on make up, look for
- ❖ Creamy concealers.
- ❖ Apply it below and above the eyelids.
- ❖ Eye shadows which are more earthy in tone.

Eyebrows

Any talk on the aesthetics of the eye is incomplete without the mention of eyebrow. Eyebrows almost dictates the character of your face. Here is how an ideal eyebrow should look like.

The Ideal Eyebrows

The eyebrow is usually divided into three portions and has to flare out at the junction of the third quarter, just above and after the pupil. The inner and beginning part of the eyebrow has to be a little lower while the outer brow has to be tapered and raised high in a flare. Observe how in older ladies the outer eyebrow becomes scanty and thin, the inner eyebrow is raised, and the lateral portion falls heavy on the eye. Therefore, a youthful eyebrow ideally should be one that is thick, dark, and where the inner side dips slightly and the outer side flares up. A good idea is to direct the beautician to do exactly that and fill in with a dark brown eye shadow with a flat eye brush instead of a black eye pencil to make it look thick and natural. You could also use some medications used for eyelash enhancement. As a home remedy, you could oil your eyebrow with coconut or castor oil and post bath, wipe your face in such a way that you direct your wet eyebrow hair upwards. You will see that instantly opens up your eyes.

As you start ageing, your eyebrows:

- Start to get scanty and thin, so you can use eyelash lengtheners like Latisse or Lashisma on your eyebrows. Some permanent tinting like tattoo can add colour. Mesotherapy with hair stimulating concoction can help as well.
- Outer corner starts to droop. This is because of the eye muscles that pull it down, so some Botox will lift it right up.
- Outer third of the eyebrow starts to dip and the fat below it regresses and the fat on the upper eyelid pulls it further down. Filler along the temple and under the tail of your brow combined with Botox helps.

- However, what you need most at any age is the shape of the brow. Here is a guide to get it right and guide your beautician to give you the shape that most compliments you. For an Indian face, the arched and the laterally flared brow suits best.
- Rub your brow hair upwards after your shower every day and see just the direction of that hair opens up your eye and illusionally lifts up your eyebrows.

Special care of your lips

You lips are the most sensual part on your face. A full, well-shaped mouth looks very attractive. Like your under-eye area, lips also have no oil glands and the skin is very thin. So dry lips are one of the first signs of ageing that you may notice. Even change in climatic conditions can make your lips look dry.

The Ideal Lips

The upper lip is more projected but less wide compared to your lower lip. It has a well-defined white role (the white raised border of the lip) along the border, the cupid's bow is well defined and the corners straight or slightly up turned. The peri-oral rhytids, meaning lines around the mouth, are also called 'smokers lines' which lead to the lipstick bleeding out. The philtral columns are the two parallel, raised lines from the central septum of nose to the cupid's bow of the upper lip and should have a slight projection to give you beautiful lips. The skin around the mouth is smooth and plump.

THE IDEAL LIPS

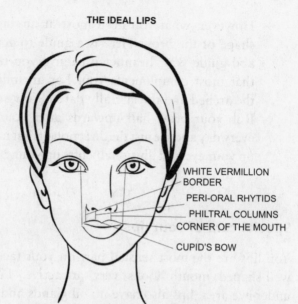

WHITE VERMILLION BORDER

PERI-ORAL RHYTIDS

PHILTRAL COLUMNS

CORNER OF THE MOUTH

CUPID'S BOW

Moisturize, moisturize, moisturize

As you grow older, your lips start getting really dry, so put a lot of cream at night. Even if you don't apply cream to your face, apply something on your lips. Post 40, even the skin around the lips starts to show signs of ageing. When applying cream on your lips, apply it a whole cm around the lips. In the morning, they will look really nice, soft, and plump. For lipstick, stick to creamy ones that make your lips look plump and soft.

Exfoliate before you hydrate

Wet your lips properly. Then move your fingers in a circular motion all over your lips to slough off the dead skin. You can even use your facial scrub to do this. Exfoliate lips every night and then apply the moisturizer.

If your lips are too dry and chapped, then apply cream at night and exfoliate in the morning. The dead skin cells will come off easily.

At your skin doctor's

There are fillers today which can be used aesthetically to make your lips look full and well-defined. You can play with the filler to just define your lip line, plump up the body of your lips, shape it up, or just hydrate without adding volume. If you've got smoker lines, then filler, Botox, and laser are good options for you.

SMACKING LIPS IS NO GOOD!

Got chapped lips? Stop licking or smacking them this instant—it will only aggravate the condition. Moreover, you will get pigmented lips and a black border around your mouth. If your lips feel dry, wash them and apply a rich cream.

Nutrition for your eyes and lips

Make sure you take enough Omega-3 fatty acids, and vitamins to get bright, beautiful eyes and lips. For many people who come to me with the problem of dark circles, I realize the problem is with the lack of elemental iron in their body, even when they are not anaemic. Check your serum ferritin and B12 levels.

A note for men

Even though you guys hate to do much for your skin, I don't think your significant other will like to kiss your chapped lips. So try and follow the lip care routine I have mentioned here. Since you are spending time in front of the mirror to heal your lips, you can do a bit extra and take care of your eyes as well. To beat tired eyes—which am sure you get after staring so long at the computer all day—use a cooling gel pack. Then apply a nice under eye cream before you get to bed.

Special care for the neck, chest, and body

Most us give step sisterly treatment to the rest of the body other than our face. There are a lot of people with well looked after faces who have hands and neck that look so much older and dull. It's such a miss match! These parts of your body are exposed to the same environmental conditions as your face. Hormones have the same effect on them as you age. So, ideally the care must remain the same. All the issues like dryness, lines, loss of fat, and pigmentation happen on all your body parts as well. Here's what you must do:

Care for you neck and chest

The quality of skin around the neck and chest is much different from the face. It is thin and collagen regeneration in this area is pretty poor. Besides, platysma, the muscles that run from your lower face to the collar bone, starts to lose tone and also pulls the skin downwards. The vertical bands become prominent and fat distribution on the lower face and neck changes. Obesity and altered thyroid and insulin levels can add to the dryness and pigmentation.

Extended care: We have a tendency to apply moisturizers, sunscreen, make up and most of our skincare regimen only up to the jawline. The best way is to make sure all your skincare practices include neck and upper chest area in their ambit. Start by keeping all these areas well moisturized. Apply moisturizers at night and keep these areas well covered to prevent sun damage. Apply sunscreen up to the neck, not just on your face. Do some stretches to help reduce fat accumulation around the neck.

You do not need separate creams for different areas. These are mostly marketing pitches. When you are using collagen stimulating cream, it's the same for every area. But if you have an oily face and dry neck skin, you may need a creamier moisturizer for the neck.

At your skin doctor's: You can also go to a doctor once in a while to get a peel or a facial, and make sure it extends up to the upper chest. This is important if you notice skin darkening around your neck and age spots appearing on your décolletage. You can use a little Botox on those vertical bands on your neck. You will immediate a fantastic tightening and a well-defined jawline. Also, you can use Botox and filler for horizontal lines as well. Mesotherapy with a very light hyaluronic acid is something which I use to give a great hydrating and tightening effect on the neck. Peels and laser might not give as good results in this area for collagen stimulation, but you can get a MesoBotox done for the bosom.

Care for your hands

Skin on your hands can get dry or dark mostly due to sun exposure. Your hands are on the wheel when you are driving, so there is greater exposure. You wash your hands most often and this rips away all the moisture. Often crinkly skin and bony tendons stand up along with the vessels on the back of the hand, making it look haggard.

Extended care: All the skincare should be extended to hands as well along with face. Always carry a rich hand moisturizing cream and apply it regularly. The scrub you use for your face can also be used for the hands. Be more receptive to night moisturizer. Also apply sunscreen regularly. Moisturize your hand every time you wash it.

At your skin doctor's: If your hands are dry and pigmented, then peels and lasers can be done. If your hands have started to look wrinkly and even bony, then you can use fillers like Juvederm which make them look more supple.

Care for your body

Dry skin, pigmentation, and stretchmarks are the most common issues that women come to me for. Like your facial skin, your body skin too gets dry. You will also notice that some areas of your body will have dark patches, especially your back and arms. Your feet also tend to look dark and dehydrated. So here's how you can deal with them.

- Change your shower gels to shower oils
- 10 min pre-bath oil massage
- Gentle exfoliation
- Moisturize on a damp body
- No harsh scrub or rubbing with towel if there is pigmentation
- Apply sunscreen on all exposed parts
- Take supplements like omega oils, multivitamins, and antioxidants

CHAPTER 12
ANTI-AGEING TREATMENTS

BEAUTY IS NOT A luck-by-chance thing. It requires diligence and hard work. Very few are really blessed with genes that retain youthful skin without much effort. For the rest there is science. Aesthetic dermatology has advanced, like in other branches of medicine, to help you look your best at every age.

The idea of 'anti-ageing' is not to freeze your face of all expressions, iron out all lines, or make skin artificially stretched and glistening. In fact, these are things you should not do! There are tools available, but the result depends on the person who wields the tool. It is like a magic wand. Just imagine if a spell were to go wrong. You'd blame the magician not the magic itself, right?

Everyone need not go to the doctor on the first sign of wrinkle and request for a Botox treatment. There are so many options available to you now that are so much more gentle and easy to do. So here I have created a list of important treatments that you can get at your doctor. I have also put down the dos and don'ts of every treatment.

To make it easy for you to understand, I have divided the various treatments into three basic types. Go ahead choose your treatment.

Simple office procedure

Takes all of 10 minutes. Can be done by a trained technician without much down time and can be repeated every 10 days to once a month as maintenance.

Medi-Facials

Medi-Facials are facials which are done under medical supervision. When you go in for a regular facial, they scrub, steam, and extract your comedones, and then apply a cream and massage for 20 minutes. Right? Have you ever asked at the salon if the extractor is sterilized? If the steam is affecting your pigmentation or not? If they are taking care to shrink the pores thereafter before applying the cream to your face? Is the massage cream suited to your skin type? Are the strokes right for your face? These are all the concerns that will be specially taken care of and individualized at an expert's clinic when you go for a Medi-Facial.

Medi-Facials that you can ask for

- Oxy-facials that use nascent, high-pressured oxygen jet to deliver vitamins into the skin. The added oxygen also has its benefits.
- Hydra facials are done with products like antioxidants and hyaluronic acid jet along with a suction.

❖ Galvanic, ultrasound facials use various equipments to drive the actives into the deeper layers of the skin.

Acid peels

It simply means applying an acid on your skin, face, or body to chemically exfoliate the top dead layer of your skin. Now what it does to your skin depends on the type of the acid, strength, layers applied, duration of application, and depth achieved.

Peels can

❖ Refresh your skin by removing the top dead layer and making it a shade lighter and brighter.
❖ Work on various types of pigmentation.
❖ Help collagen regeneration, thus working on fine lines, skin texture, scars etc.
❖ Heal your acne.
❖ Increase the penetration of other actives by doing away with the barrier—dead skin.

Microdermabrasion

Popularly called skin polishing. It is a physical exfoliating treatment. It could be done just with abrasive specks of diamond on the tip of a suction apparatus. Or continuous aluminium micro crystals hit your skin and scrape the top layer which is sucked back through a vacuum method. In my clinic, I do not use this on the face at all. We only use this on the body skin as I know there are better, gentler, and newer ways to achieve the same result on your facial skin.

Skin polishing can be done
- ❖ On skin sensitive to peels.
- ❖ To get the dead layer out so the other actives are better absorbed.
- ❖ Deep pore cleansing.
- ❖ Before certain lasers.

A note of caution

BEFORE THE TREATMENT

- ❖ Prep your skin with hydroquinone and other skin lighteners to avoid pigmentation if deep peels are to be done.
- ❖ Hydrate and moisturize your skin well.
- ❖ Inform your doctor if your skin feels sensitive and dry.

AFTER THE TREATMENT

- ❖ Avoid the sun for the next 24 hours.
- ❖ No harsh active ingredients in your day and night cream that is acids, peroxide, and anti-ageing.
- ❖ Further exfoliation at home.

Equipment-based procedure

Not all equipments at your doctor's office are lasers. Depending on the technology that is used, it could be laser, lights, radio frequency, ultrasound, and infrared.

Laser

Lasers are of different kinds. The type of laser used on you depends on the specific problem that needs to be addressed. Your doctor is the best judge in choosing the type. Lasers do not understand skin, hair, or blood.They only work on colour or pigment. However, there are some that work with water in your tissue as their target.

Then there are different ways of delivering the beam to your skin. So your doctor can work with full beam, fractionated, or pixelated so it's not bulk heating which leads to the unwanted effects of a laser. Depending on how much time is taken to pass the given beam, it could be long pulsed, or Q-switched. It could be ablative or non-ablative depending on whether it burns off a portion of your skin or just works with it intact.

These can be administered by a qualified technician after a doctor's consent. Different doctors do it differently. In my practice I do it all myself. Others choose to set the parameters and have the technician perform the treatment. Most of these have to be repeated multiple times to achieve results. You will also have to go for maintenance sessions later at certain intervals.

Laser can be used:

- ❖ For collagen stimulation to improve skin texture, thickness, scars, pores etc.
- ❖ To treat pigmentation problems like dark circles, tattoo, post-inflammatory, post acne, freckles, age spots, and tan. However, some conditions like melasma do not really respond well. The marks may even get darker on a rebound, so be careful.
- ❖ For fat reduction. You can reduce cellulite and get spot weight reduction through a combination of various technologies like deep tissue massage, infrared, radio frequency, and ultrasound—all

causing deep tissue heating. You can also try the newer fat freezing equipment.

+ For wiping away scars, a combination of lasers and radio frequency with micro needling are all a good bet to choose from.

+ Treat broken capillaries. A combination of lasers and radio frequency works wonderfully.

A note of caution

BEFORE THE TREATMENT

+ Be careful in choosing your doctor and centre. Make sure the equipments are FDA approved and not substandard Asian knockoffs.

+ No tanning before treatment.

+ No active infection or open wound.

AFTER THE TREATMENT

+ Appropriate cooling for certain lasers.

+ You might get burns after a hair reduction treatment since the diode laser used is in close contact with skin.

+ Hypo pigmentation becomes a problem for some, especially those who tend to show healing with skin that is lighter in colour. This generally goes away after a few months.

+ Sunscreen and healing creams.

+ Avoid sun exposure.

+ No swimming to avoid sun and chlorine.

Microneedling

Multiple tiny needles are poked together into your skin to achieve a wound depth of anywhere between 0.5 mm to 3 mm. This stimulates collagen and drives the active products in to help repair and restore the skin further.

How does this work? Brain perceives these tiny needle injuries as any other injury. So it immediately starts the tissue repair process by stimulating the collagen. So this is a very pocket friendly option to laser if you want simple solution to acne scar, anti-ageing or even a dose of a skin brightening vitamin. It can be administered through disposable derma rollers or the doctor could also use stamps of multiple needles on an automated equipment. I have found great results when I have combined micro needling with radio frequency.

Injectable

These are procedures performed with a needle and syringe. When done right, the results are magical. These can be used to erase fine lines, lighten and tighten skin, and even contour facial features. The popular injectables are:

Botox

A protein that relaxes the muscle underneath your skin, so the lines on them relax.

Filler

A volumizer when placed in appropriate layers of your face can either fill in deep lines, or hollows like the under eye and temple; fill to lift the cheek and the brow, fill to contour your cheek and chin. For me it is a great sculpting tool, without actually holding a knife. It is an inert substance and slowly degraded by the body, so the results can stay from anywhere between 6 months to a couple of years.

What is the difference between botox and filler?

It's amusing that most people think Botox and filler are two solutions that one can choose from to address the same issue! NO. Here is the difference:

BOTOX

What: Botox is a protein which relaxes the muscle to which it is injected. The doctor decides the dose after examining and taking into consideration various indicators.

Why and where: It is usually used for active wrinkles, i.e. lines that come on expression. But the newer indication are towards reshaping like in the jaw, reducing the downward tug of the facial muscles like the ones on the neck or the ones that pull your brow down, functional correction like bunny smile or flared nostrils, or for general health and well-being benefits like treating migraine or excessive sweating.

How long: procedure should take no more than 10 minutes. The result is temporary, lasts 3 to 4 months, depending on the dose and site may vary a bit more. The result takes anywhere between 3 to 10 days to be visible.

For more information on Botox, you can look at this video on my website: http://www.drrashmishetty.com/pages/botox.html

FILLER

What: Filler is a biological gel of varying consistency and composition.

Why and Where: This is injected to the area of deficit; passive lines (lines that show up even when the face is at rest) like the laugh lines, deep set frown lines etc., volume loss like in mid cheek or under eye, facial enhancement like lip/chin/cheek augmentation, any scars; or for hydration, skin refreshing, fine static lines as well.

How long: Depending on the complexity of the area or work, it may take anywhere between 5 to 20 minutes. It lasts between 6 months to 2 years, and maybe even more varying from person to person. Repeated treatments tend to last longer. The result is instant!

For more information on filler, you can look at this video on my website: http://www.drrashmishetty.com/pages/filler.html

So basically they do different jobs, which complement each other. In a few situations like crow's feet, frown lines, puckered chin , smoker's lines around your mouth—they kind of can be used either/or and even together to get better and long lasting results.

The magic is in the doctor's skill and the time most spent is on assessment + planing the treatment.

Mesotherapy

Can be used to deliver different substances—depending on what one wants to achieve— into the skin. It can be used for skin tightening, hydration, lightening, and to treat severe hair fall and hair thinning on the scalp. The areas to be treated are all injected in tiny amounts with tiny needles into the mesodermis—one of the deeper layers of the skin.

Lipo dissolve

Substances like phospodylcholene, L-carnitine are used to burn fat in a spot of area. I inject this right at the pocket of fat that you may want to melt. It is a great sculpting method for the body. It can be used to reduce love handles, slim down lower abdomen, thighs, or even the fat on your too-rounded cheeks.

While Botox and fillers are usually one-time treatments that give you the desired results, the other injectables require multiple sessions. However, know that none of the treatments can give you permanent results, so you need to get them done again at set intervals.

What happens if you do not wish to do these treatments anymore?

Any of these treatments always leaves you feeling better and enhanced, even if the best result wears off with time. But you never go worse from your starting point. So even if you want to try them once, or want to pamper yourself for an occasion, go right ahead.

What can go wrong?

Your face could freeze!
    You could look like someone else!
    You could end up like a chipmunk!
    You could look a little too 'done'.

Okay, calm down. All this 'can happen' but need not happen. Go to the right doctor. It is the aesthetic sense of the doctor that counts. We all study the same science as doctors, but it is how the doctor wields the tools of beauty that counts. In our line of aesthetic cosmetology, the doctor is an artist. Work should be done in such a way that everybody compliments you about your fresh face and beauty but keeps wondering what's your secret.

For more detailed information on various forms of treatment, please visit my website http://www.drrashmishetty.com/

Make up that takes five years off your face

- ❖ A good primer that corrects the oil or dry excess from the skin.
- ❖ The right shade of base that conceals all the flaws in your tone.
- ❖ A highlighter on the cheek bone and the temples and upper eyelid just below the eyebrow, forehead, near the hair line and chin.
- ❖ Work on one of your best features—the eye or lip.
- ❖ Eyebrows and eyelashes are the most important, even if you want a no make up look or simply no make up at all. Hydration, sunscreen, and eyebrow and eyelash tint and face looks fresh and youthful.
- ❖ Do not forget the upper eye lid and neck when you do the base.

Age aggressors

A few things that have definite downward effect on beauty and ageing and that you can very well live without are

Sugar: As I mentioned in the chapter on skin and hair care during the festive season, sugar, in all of its forms— high fructose corn syrup, cane sugar—suppresses the activity of our white blood cells and so makes you more susceptible to colds, flu, and worsens allergies. It breaks down good proteins, leading to advanced glycation end products (AGE). AGE makes the proteins in the collagen and hair stiff and hard; thus speeding up the skin ageing and making hair brittle, and therefore it is one of the main contributors to wrinkles, deep lines, and sagging skin. When our blood sugar and insulin levels rise, whether from dietary sugar, starchy foods, or from stress, we experience a serious increase in inflammatory chemicals. This causes acne to worsen dramatically along with Cortisol and other adrenal steroids that stimulate the sebaceous (oil) glands.

So overloading on high sugar foods in the name of desserts or a spoon of sugar in your daily tea, or our great Indian weddings and festivals which are round the year, causes damage to your skin and hair.

My suggestion is be mindful of what you are eating all the time. Alpha lipoid acid is one of the best to combat AGE, whether eaten or applied. Instead you can take in natural sugars found in fruits and vegetables which are high in anti-inflammatory antioxidants.

Salt: Excessive salt in your body increases all sorts of inflammation and retains fluid everywhere. The swollen joints, breasts, and belly are partly because of fluid retention aggravated by salt. Ayurvedic doctors say that your joint pains and systemic illnesses can be helped with a no salt diet. For us now think swollen face and puffy eyes! So NO salt, especially post sunset, because salt makes you retain water. So if you have puffy eyes early in the morning, or a water retained feeling on the bust and belly areas, then the easy and best trick will be to cut down on your salt intake in the second half of your day.

Smoke: Smoke and pollution damages hair and skin. You will find your hair feeling dry and scalp irritated and even itchy. Too much exposure can lead to boils/folliculitis, skin rash, and acne exacerbation. Wearing a scarf and braiding your hair will prevent it from harmful smoke. But the smoke that you drag into your system is the most harmful. Smoking pretty much does to your skin from inside what sun does from the outside—it makes your collagen weak, skin look tired, interferes with your blood supply, and slows down wound healing. I always tell my patients that drinking alcohol once in moderation is okay but smoking is an absolute no!

Alcohol: Alcohol adds to your woes! What is left of your skin and hair will be done to with alcohol. It makes the skin flushed with broken capillaries and dehydration. Alcohol is okay in moderation, but flood your system with water after you indulge in drinking.

Skimping on your sunscreen: I have told you all through my book how sun harms your skin and how important sunscreen is. Now if you take a very little quantity, the size of a bitter pill, it's not going to help. You actually need a dollop, about 2 big pea size, for your face alone to even come near to achieving the SPF protection mentioned on the tube.

Using the wrong cleanser: It can strip all your moisture, making your skin further dry and increasing the fine lines, irritating the area around the eye and mouth. So go for a creamy cleanser.

Overeating: When you gain a lot of weight, you know what happens to the skin—it gets mottled and flushed. And then when you lose weight, stretch marks and sagging appears. Yes, there are creams and oils and lasers and peels and radio frequency and micro needling. But even when we put them all together, we can't get back your skin 'just right'. But the issue I want to highlight is—post 40 how will you lose it? I have been 49 kg since I started getting on the scale and today at 40 and mom of a teen, I still am 49. The difference is I could eat a lion's share and stay that way earlier but ever since I touched 40, everything changed. Now I cast a fleeting glimpse at greasy, carb-ridden food and walk away.

Sleeping positions: Be mindful of your sleeping positions. Always sleep on your back. Compressing your face against the pillow will cause more creases, alter facial shape, and cause acne.

Facial expressions: Keep repeating only the happy ones. Sad ones stick on too.

You know your skin is undergoing premature ageing due to UV rays when:

* You notice fine wrinkles around the eyes and mouth, and frown lines on the forehead.
* You see spider veins on the nose, cheeks, and neck.
* Various pigmented spots such as freckles, solar lentigines (known as age or liver spots, although they are unrelated to the liver), and an uneven skin colour.
* A general loss of skin tone in sun exposed areas.
* Taut lips that start to lose some colour and fullness. Lips look drawn, pale, and thin, and lose some definition. There may even be scaling.
* The skin feels leathery and sags.
* Broken blood vessels on the nose and cheeks are often visible.
* Red, rough, scaly spots, called Actinic (sun-related) Keratoses, may appear. These may be pre-cancerous and require treatment.
* Increased sensitivity and skin redness.

CHAPTER 13

READING BEAUTY PRODUCT LABELS LIKE AN EXPERT

WE ARE SURROUNDED BY a plethora of beauty products—sunscreen lotions, skin lightening creams, anti-ageing creams and capsules, moisturizing lotions, and many more. They have evolved a great deal in terms of sensory, active ingredients, and variety in terms of getting more skin specific. But for you to pick the right one can be a nightmare.

A simple way is to go by:

- ❖ The amount you want to spend; that narrows a lot down.
- ❖ A reputed company. They do their research well and stand by their claims mostly.
- ❖ Your skin goal and your top priority, whether it is skin lightening, anti-ageing, or sun protection. Most products nowadays cater to all of these.
- ❖ Your skin type—every standard company has this mentioned(Oil/dry/dehydrated/sensitive/damaged/acne prone/anti-ageing etc).

This narrows down your choice to the minimum.

Now here's some more gyan to follow while while you go beauty shopping.

#1 – Reading the label

'The label' is a window to what your product is and what it can do. It has enough information to guide you to pick the right product that suits your skin in terms of skin type and beauty goal.

Usually the label at the back of the bottle has a lot of information starting from the ingredient list, the skin type it is most suitable for, the application instructions, a warning sign, the date and place of manufacturing, the expiry date, and a lot more.

Make sure you look for the following on a bottle/tube label:

Skin type: Very essential. Be assured that the product suits your skin type—dry, normal, or oily. This is always specified on the bottle, mostly for sunscreens, cleansers, face washes, and night and day creams. For the rest, you need to seek expert advice.

Pictorial description of the ingredients: It is a trend now to have a small pictures of the main ingredients shown on the front side of the bottle with the description of that ingredient carried to the back of the bottle. These are usually called the 'active ingredients' which are the ones that really bring out the action intended by the product. Sometimes the common/familiar name is used—like turmeric, rose—but at times you have scientific names like curcumin i.e. turmeric or Peucedanum Graveolens extract which is actually 'dill extract'.

Sometimes you find a pamphlet given along with the bottle which carries enough information about the active ingredients.

Directions for usage: Always remember too much usage and too little usage of the product will not give the expected results. The right amount should be used to get the right results. One fingertip unit is approximately 0.5-1gm.

Warning: It simply states which areas should be avoided so that no unnecessary reaction occurs. Mostly it is sensitive areas or areas with thinner skin like the under eye, corner of your mouth, crease of your nose etc. Sometimes, even to avoid the sun exposed areas or simply sensitive areas, you must read the warning so as to avoid using it on skin areas that are extra dry, red, irritated, or flaky.

Source of product: Some products contain materials from animal sources which is clearly mentioned on the label. An easy way is to look out for a red dot for animal source and green dot for plant source in a black square on one of the corners of the packaging. Animal tested: Usually clinical trials are conducted on animals to check the safety of the products. If the product has gone through animal testing, it is usually mentioned on the label. By and large, there is no animal testing now as there are a lot of other methods available. For example, digitizing skin replica can be a reliable method for wrinkle assessment and so can be used before and after may be 60 or 90 days of a particular portion or ingredient.

Colour of the product: The colour is always mentioned on the product, so ensure that the colour is the same once you open the bottle/tube. Some lotions and portions can be oxidized by the sun. For example, notice how vitamin C creams come in a black jar or a completely opaque jar to cut out light and UV damage completely. So it is important for you to make a mental note of the colour of the product you use.

Manufacturing and the expiry date: This indicates how long a product is considered good to use under normal conditions of storage and use depending on the date it has been packaged/manufactured. Cosmeceuticals, i.e. cosmetic creams with actives not of medical grade, do not usually have an expiry date. They are good to use for up to 3 years after the manufacturing. However, if there is an active ingredient like an anti-acne or pigmentation cream of a medical grade or 'as per doctor's prescription' written on it, then it usually is 2 years. Or you can simply look at the expiry date on the pack. I have a practice of asking my patients to get all their previous skincare products during my first consultation with them. I see that the jars are not really in a state that it is supposed to be in—the tubes are twisted and pealed, the creams are leaking out of the jars and nozzles. Mostly we use hands to dig in from open jars, so I'd say throw them out after a year. And anyway if you are using the right quantities, with the quantities that are packaged, no face care lotion should last for more than 6 months. So my expiry date for all face care products is 1 year.

Clinically proven: This means it has been proven to work in clinical tests or in a clinical environment.

Temperature: Extremely necessary to follow to ensure that the product remains in its perfect state without giving off a bad colour, odour, and it must keep the actives active. Products are best kept at 20 degree centigrade, but this may not always be possible, so be mindful of your creams in terms of colour and consistency.

#2 – What's in the bottle?

To know what's in a bottle of the beauty potion that you have picked up, just scan down to the 'ingredients'. Don't get overwhelmed by the seeming jargon listed there.

Know that usually the ingredients in highest amounts or concentrations in the potion are written first followed by the next set of important ingredients. Near the end of the list you might find out about the preservatives used. There is always the base formulation or stabilizing agents into which the active ingredients are added. Sometimes you will also notice that the publicised active is listed way down on the list. That is mostly because the concentration of the active used is less, which does not necessarily mean that the product is any less effective.

Creams/lotions/serums: What's all the fuss about?

It is all about oil-in-water or water-in-oil emulsion, oil-in-water being the non-sticky, non greasy one and water-in-oil being the heavy one (usually the night creams).

Even though serums seem to have grabbed all the limelight of late, they are nothing but water-in- silicone/ oil-in-silicon + oils, i.e. generally low viscosity translucent liquids. These are light and presumed as more potent than creams or as concentrates. But that's a marketing strategy. All they are is a different medium and silicon gives you the sense of a velvet finish.

Here goes the list:-

Peptides: These could be the pentapeptides, oligopeptides, tripeptides, tetrapeptides—all of these actually help in the reduction of wrinkles and facial lines. These help stimulate collagen synthesis.

Peptides are amino acids linked up in short chains. These were originally developed as a part of wound healing research on human fibro blasts, i.e. cells that produce new cells. Basically 3 types are used in cosmetic creams and portions—signal peptides, carrier peptides, and neurotransmitter modulating peptides.

Peptides in general help stimulate fibroblast production, down regulate the elastin and collagen degrading factors. Also increases feedback regulation of new collagen synthesis. .

Carrier peptides stabilize and deliver some heavy molecules like metals and trace elements in your creams.

Neurotransmitter modulating ones are what the 'Botox creams' have in them.

TREATMENT ACTIVES:

➤ Antioxidants: This skin boosting complex will have a blend of:
✤ Vitamin A/retinoids: These are a group of compounds that have the basic core structure of vitamin A. It is available as oxidized metabolites

and now synthetically developed ones like tretinoin, adapalene etc. In the synthetic forms, the irritation factor which otherwise a retin A causes is lesser. The benefits in whichever form are protection from photo damaged skin, ageing skin, acne and more serious issues like psoriasis.

❖ Vitamin E: Also called tocopherol acetate, an antioxidant that protects the cells from the damaging effects of oxidation, helps in some pigmentary and dry skin conditions. Some antioxidants like glutathione or ubiquinol can be synthesised by us. Vitamin E has to be supplemented.

❖ Vitamin C: Ascorbic acid, ascorbylglucoside acts as a naturally occurring antioxidant essential for collagen synthesis. It adds on to the antioxidant action of vitamin E and lightens pigmentation. It also reduces the elastin accumulation in photoaged skin (thick rubbery feeling/looking skin). Vitamin C is poorly absorbed when taken orally. It is therefore most popular in application forms. If your Vit c is turning yellow, then the active form L ascorbic acid is used. Therefore, in the recent formulations, there might be magnesium ascorbyl phosphate and ascorbylpalmitate. These are more stable. Even on topical application, it enhances collagen production and reduces collagen breakdown. Also great to protect you from the oxidative damage caused by the sun. Therefore, I recommend all my patients to apply a layer of vitamin C and then top it with sunscreen as sunscreen alone cannot stop the free radical damage caused by UV rays. It has an anti-inflammatory property. Inflammation, it has been proved, leads to most unwanted changes in the body, inside out .

+ Vitamin B
+ B-3 Niacinamide: Prevents photodamage, helps in skin redness like in rosacea by reducing factors causing skin irritation, atopic (allergic) skin types by reducing water loss from the skin. Niacinamide has been one of the most popular skin lightening ingredients used in over-the-counter skin lightening creams by reducing the transfer and production of melanin—the pigment that causes darkening. Also prevents yellowing of skin, so it is popular among the fair but yellow under tone skins like in Japan and Far Eastern countries. It helps improve texture, pore size, and decreases the excess oil in the skin.
+ B5- Panthenol: Mainly used in treating bruises, scars, burns etc. It promotes cell multiplication, stimulates growth, and increases skin lipid production. It is cosmetically used for hydration and repair of skin.

ANTI-AGEING INGREDIENTS

> Vitamin A derivatives:
+ Retinyl Palmitate: A derivative of vitamin A, helps stimulate collagen and reverses the signs of prematurely-induced photoageing. Helps to increase skin elasticity while enhancing water barrier properties.
+ Retinyl Proprionate: Retinoids are natural or synthetic substances derived from vitamin A. Clinical studies have proven that the topical

application of retinyl proprionate, a less irritating form of vitamin A used for conditioning, is effective in reducing the appearance of fine lines and wrinkles. It also smoothens skin texture and reduces the look of discoloration.

- ✤ Peptides: improves the appearance of skin ageing without the irritation caused by retinoids. These are short-chained proteins which stimulate production of new collagen and elastin and also decrease collagen breakdown. The neurotransmitter modulating peptides are the ingredients in the 'Botox creams'. They act on the neurotransmitters interface between the nerve and the muscle contraction .

- ➤ Hyaluronic acid/propylene glycol/glycerine: Humectants that help retain skin moisture.

- ➤ AHA or Alpha hydroxy acid: For exfoliating skin cells and resurfacing newer layer.

- ✤ Glycolic acid: Mainly used to improve the appearance and texture of the skin by a 'peel action', helps improve acne scarring, hyper pigmentation, age spots, and wrinkles.

- ✤ Lactic acid: Helps retexture skin's surface and stimulates cell renewal and cell turnover, helps control melanin synthesis, hydrates skin, and stimulates ceramide production.

- ➤ BHA or Beta hydroxy acid: One form of BHA is Salicylic Acid which acts as an effective keratolytic (exfoliant) agent, also an anti-irritant, and functions mainly as an anti-inflammatory agent. It encourages the exfoliation of dead skin and renews the outer layer of skin.

SKIN LIGHTENING AGENTS

> ➢ Kojic acid: It is a by-product of the fermentation process of malting rice for use in the manufacture of sake(Japanese rice wine); it is effective for inhibiting melanin production, helps in skin lightening and establishing an even skin tone.

> ➢ Hydroquinone: It is the primary topical ingredient for inhibiting melanin production. Helps in reducing and potentially eliminating brown spots and hyperpigmentation from melasma.

> ➢ Arbutin: derived from bearberry. Less effective than kojic

> ➢ Vitamin C: interferes with pigment production.

> ➢ Niacinamide: It is one of the safest skin-lightening agents and the commonest ingredients in your over-the-counter product.

> ➢ Azelaic acid: natural ingredient. Highly active on pigmented skin. Apply twice daily. This is one of my favourite ingredients.

> ➢ Liquorice root: Interrupts the stimulation of an enzyme that activates melanin production, works on lightening dark spots and hyper pigmentation.

> ➢ Botanical anti inflammatories and soothing agents: Ginkgo biloba, green tea, allantoin; mostly used in eye creams: witch hazel, green tea; mostly in products for acne prone skin, aloe vera; this will be the species with the medicinal properties. There are more than 400 species and only a countable few have the medicinal property and after plucking, if it is not preserved well, the benefit is soon gone. This one is for all of you who think it is okay to

pot it, pluck it, and use it. Also naturals do not mean no allergies/no harm.

➤ Some of the most recent used herbs and botanicals in skin and hair care are the ones that our Indian families have told us all this while like garlic, turmeric, basil, almond, neem, sunflower, pomegranate, teas, milk extracts, and hibiscus.

➤ Citrus Grandis or Grapefruit Extract: Rich in flavonoids that inhibit Tyrosinase; a natural source of vitamin C that inhibits melanogenesis.

METALS

Zinc: Helps in cell repair and growth, fights sun damage.

Copper: Collagen formation and hair growth and strength.

Iron: Apart from all the other benefits to health, it is very important for skin glow and oxygenation. An iron deficiency leads to hair fall and dark circles around the eyes.

Aluminium: Used in antiperspirants.

Magnesium: Maintains skin health.

Calcium: Cell growth and anti-inflammation.

Silver: Anti-bacterial.

SUN BLOCKS

➤ Avobenzene: Which absorb the UV radiations.
➤ Octinoxate/Octisalate/Octocrylene/Homosalate/Oxybenzone: Broad spectrum sunscreen.
➤ Titanium oxide: Offers broad spectrum sun protection, physical sunscreen/texturizer.

> ➤ Zinc oxide: Physical sunscreen with soothing properties. These physical ones block light and are the ones that give you the white colour on the skin while you apply sunscreen. In a paste form you'll see sportsmen using this to protect their skin from UV damage.

MOISTURIZERS

1. Occlusive components: They slow down the water loss by evaporation—more like moisture sealants like oils/waxes, petrolatum, mineral oils, paraffin, squalene, silicone derivatives, fatty acids, wax esters. These are best used when there is some moisture to start with, not when the skin is super dry already. So either you use them on wet/damp skin or use a mist to hydrate the skin and then use these agents.

2. Humectants: They attract water from your skin or the atmosphere. These include glycerine, urea, and sodium lactate. So it's not a good idea to use them when the ambient humidity is low.

3. Emollients: These are oils that give a soothing feeling on dry skin like castor oil, jojoba oil, coconut oil, glyceryl and coctyl stearate.

FEW COMMONS

Glycerin: A humectant that helps hold moisture.

Oils: Like coconut oil/almond oil that soften and smoothen the skin.

Cera alba/beeswax: Softens and smoothens the skin. Also contains vitamin A which may be beneficial in softening and rehydrating dry skin and in cell reconstruction.

Shea butter: A rich fruit-based moisturizer that also has vitamin A to soothe dryness caused in mature skin.

3 – Know the jargon

There are these set of terms that you see on almost all the products that your buy, but you are confused as what they really mean. Not knowing their meaning can lead you to buying the wrong product or formulation. So what do they mean? Read on to find out.

Inactive ingredients: These could be preservatives, colours, fragrance, or flavours used in the making of the product and which do not necessarily contribute to the function/effect that the product claims.

Non-comedogenic: Cosmetic products that are non-comedogenic (or referred to as non-occlusive) don't plug the pores, so don't cause skin irritation or pimples.

Parabens: Preservatives in cosmetics.

SPF: SPF is an acronym for sun protection factor. Sunscreen products have an SPF; the higher the SPF, the more protection you get from sunburn. 1 SPF gives a 10-minute protection under the sun.

TPI: TPI stands for tan protection index .Simply put, it is the number of minutes you are in the sun and will not get tanned. This is denoted by the plus signs on the bottle.

Sunblock: Sunblock, as opposed to sunscreen which acts more like a UV filter, is a lotion that actually blocks the UV-rays. Mostly these are physical blocks which hold the sunscreen like a fabric or metal shield.

Male grooming: Is it any different?

Back in the days, my staff would giggle if an occasional male patient came to the clinic. Today, male grooming is the norm. In fact, almost 30% of my patients are males. And why not? Men are now open to grooming and bold in their choices in order to look their best. Their hair is still their main concern. However, skin sagging, ageing, and pigmentation are slowly becoming other key skin concerns. The skincare product providers have also seen a great potential in the male grooming market and are therefore coming out with specific male skincare ranges to suit their skin and lifestyle. So what is it that makes the male and female cosmetic products different? And is there really any difference in the first place?

For starters, let us understand the skin structure:

The skin is basically a layered structure which is the same in a man and a woman. The difference simply lies in that male and female skins differ in hormone metabolism, hair growth pattern, the sweat rate, production of sebum, surface pH, and fat accumulation.

Male skin is approximately 20% thicker than female skin. Men have a higher percentage of elastin and collagen. Women have a thicker layer of subcutaneous fat than men but men have more collagen and lose collagen at a slower rate than women when past middle age.

Males sweat more, produce more sebum, and are more prone to develop alopecia (hair loss) and acne. As males sweat more, it creates an environment conducive for bacterial growth which results in the production of odour (one of the reasons why male cosmetic products have a stronger fragrance). Males tend to have more body hair which is also thicker and which gives a higher body surface area for bacterial colonization. Thus, the popularity for antibacterial soaps for men.

Considering these differences, the market is flooded with 'Gendered cosmetic products' which are designed keeping in mind these differences promising maximum benefit when one uses them for a specific purpose.

The most commonly demanded cosmetic range by the males are:

- ❖ Moisturizers: Because regular usage of razors results in dry skin.
- ❖ Beard oils and conditioners: To soften not only the beard hair but also the skin underneath.
- ❖ Aftershave lotions: To soften and smoothen the skin.
- ❖ Sunscreen lotion/creams: Sun protection from tanning and pigmentation.
- ❖ Skin lightening/fairness creams
- ❖ Anti-ageing creams: To fade out the fine lines, crow's feet, and smile lines

How are they special for men

1. Fragrance: Body odour is stronger in men, thereby the need for a stronger fragrance in the products— lotions, body creams etc. Females prefer a flowery/ sweet smelling cream or lotion as against a male who would prefer a stronger fragrance.

2. Packaging: The bottle/tubes have a more strong look, a geometric shape as compared to the female cosmetic product packaging in terms of colour, images, graphics, and shape.

3. Habit: Women are more emotional in terms of their purchasing habits whereas men are more technical and functional. Men look for products that will give them results.

5. Ingredients: Men prefer products which are invisible, quickly penetrable, easy to use, less process-oriented, pleasant to put, less fragrant, and have a visible effect. The ingredients thus used would be modified as compared to a female product but would be the same type of ingredients. Like the alcohol content could be higher to give a cooler after feel which would not be necessarily needed for a woman. Men prefer creams that seep in rapidly. Thus they generally prefer a lightweight cream or a serum whereas a woman would apply a thick/rich creamy lotion which would leave a velvety after feel.

   The ingredients are the same, the difference lies in the composition and the requirement.

5. Requirements: The difference in the cosmetic products is also based on requirements. Like, men

need aftershave lotions to keep their skin smooth
and beard conditioners to keep the beard soft.

6. Skin Functionality: TEWL (Trans-epidermal water
loss) is the epidermal barrier which is weaker in men
as compared to females. Studies have shown that
testosterone can have negative effects on epidermal
barrier function. Men's skincare must therefore be
formulated to assist the skin repair itself and protect
the integrity of the epidermal barrier layer.

There are a variety of gendered cosmetic products
available in the market but basically the male and female
cosmetic products are made to serve the same purpose—
either to cleanse or moisturize the skin, protect from sun,
or reduce wrinkles. They differ mainly in the aesthetic
sense and appeal. One could use or exchange products
but this should be done only if the product serves your
purpose and suits your skin type.

Too high a concentration of either ingredient should
not affect your skin. For example, a female having dry
skin will benefit from using a heavy moisturizer while
the same used by a male could result in an acne outbreak
(male skin is considered to be more oily).

Refrain from switching to another product if your
current product suits your skin need. Whatever product
you choose, select wisely and continue using it for
maximum results! In case of a doubt, consult your skin
doctor as he/she can correctly guide you in selecting
wisely. For as we know our skin is a mirror that reflects
radiance if well taken care of, so go ahead and PAMPER
it smartly and correctly.

CHAPTER 14

GOODIES FOR GREAT SKIN

FOR THE CONCLUDING CHAPTER of the book, I have taken help from experts in the field of fitness, health, and nutrition to help you achieve the skin you always wanted. From tips on looking forever young—Hollywood style—by renowned dermatologist Ava Shamban MD; benefits of a focussed workout and how it works wonders for your skin by Shalini Bhargava; lip-smacking anti-ageing food recipes by Suman Agarwal to simple do-it-yourself home remedies for beautiful skin by Arundhathi and the impact of ageing on a woman's mind by Dr Anjali Chhabria—this chapter contains all the goodies one could want for great skin. So read on and try to make the best use of the wisdom of these experts.

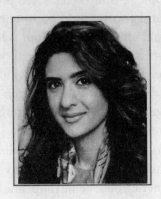

POOJA MAKHIJA,
NUTRITIONIST, CLINICAL DIETICIAN, AND
CELEBRITY FOOD GURU

I still remember the first day I met her—a pretty-looking girl clutching onto the laptop her father-in-law had gifted you. We started our careers together and we've become, if I may say so, 'celebrities' in our respective fields. Thank god for our genes. We're slim and have great skin and we have a giggle when people meet us and often think it's our handy job on each other :). Thanks a ton for being a part of my book.

Five anti-ageing tips for forever young skin

1. Youth preserving food best known to man is in the form of Omega-3 fatty-acids. To procure this in its most natural form would be to consume fatty fish like salmon, mackerel, or tuna. Other foods rich in these are almonds, soya, olive oil, and ricebran oil. Flaxseeds and flax seed oil is also an excellent source of this EFA; it is also rich in phytoestrogens which have a synergistic effect along with Omega-3 to give you young, youthful skin.

2. Glowing healthy skin is a reflection of a balanced well-nourished body. Adequate hydration and an antioxidant rich diet, being the prime focus. To ensure your daily dose of epidermal enhancing vitamins, you must include a tall glass of freshly prepared veggie juice. Include carrots (vitamin A rich), tomatoes (lycopene and vitamin C rich), avocados (Essential fatty acids (EFA) and vitamin E rich), parsley (chlorophyll, vitamin B12, Folic acid rich)

3. Green tea: it is rich in flavonoids which help protect skin against acne, pigmentations, or wrinkles. Probiotic yogurt is very important for healthy skin because it improves your immune system and kills bacteria that cause acne and other skin problems like psorasis.

4. Natural vitamins and minerals are collagen's best friend. Egg whites are a strong source of zinc, an essential vitamin that keeps skin firm and youthful. Pomegranates are loaded with nutrients including polyphenols, a very potent antioxidant which is best known to boost collagen.

5. **Last but the best!**

   Vegetable juice is the easiest, healthiest, and yummiest way to nourish your body with skin-enhancing, tresses-strengthening, anti-ageing, antioxidant rich vitamins and minerals.

   ❖ Unlike fruit juices, which spike your sugar levels, vegetable juices provide a concentrated burst of glorious vitamins and antioxidants. Make your own with the help of the following steps:

   ❖ **Wash all vegetables thoroughly.** A final rinse with potassium permanganate is also recommended.

   ❖ **Choose a minimum of 3 different vegetables** (preferably of 3 different colours so that you get a host of vitamins and minerals) Peel and cut vegetables and put them in a mixer (not in a juicer, as juicers require more vegetables).

   ❖ **Add water:** the juice should be a combination of water and vegetables in about the same proportion.

   ❖ **Blend and strain** the juice into a glass.

   ❖ **Take 50 per cent of the roughage** (pulp that you have taken out) and put it back into the glass.

   ❖ **Add some flavouring or seasoning** if you like (rock salt, pepper, fresh ginger).

   ❖ **Drink up** immediately! (Don't wait for too long as exposure to air reduces the juice's nutritional value)

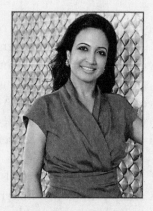

SUMAN AGARWAL,
NUTRITIONIST AND FITNESS CONSULTANT

I met Suman at a talk show where both of us were invited as expert speakers. It was at the event that I first listened to her talk about recipes with rapt attention and decided I needed to have her contribute to my book. Thank you so much for readily writing in.

Anti-ageing food recipes

Ageing is a natural process which we cannot stop, but we can slow this process down by eating healthy. So why not join the trend of eating anti-ageing foods and age beautifully?

The basic essential nutrients for our body that need to be taken in a balanced manner include carbohydrates, protein, and fats. Out of these, **proteins and fats are the most** important for weight management, anti-ageing, and immunity. Protein can be obtained from vegetarian sources like pulses, tofu, milk, and curd and non-vegetarian sources like chicken, fish, and eggs. Red meat is avoidable. High fibre foods are very important to have a blemish-free skin, reduce bad cholesterol, and protect your heart. Include more fibre in your diet (e.g. oats). Include 8-10 servings of vegetables and 2-3 servings of fruit to your diet. If your heart is healthy and is working in good capacity, it will show on your face.

Here are some anti-ageing foods that will help you look beautiful and stay healthy.

1. Youthful Yogurt

It's a part of everyday Indian diet which has many good qualities. Being rich in proteins, calcium, and vitamins it tops the list of anti-ageing foods. It will not just give you better muscle and bone strength, it will also improve your immunity and in turn help you to fight immune related diseases. Yogurt acts as probiotic and helps stomach digest food better.

2. Beautiful Berries

Berries themselves look delicious and beautiful and do the same to our body by giving us the required antioxidants and vitamin C which helps in reducing the free radicals and prevent cell damage and reduce inflammation.

3. Longevity leafy vegetables

Studies have shown that green leafy vegetables increase our longevity as they are rich in beta carotenes, vitamins, and fibre that are heart friendly and keep the blood pressure in control.

4. Crunchy nuts

Nuts not only add texture to our foods but give us the best unsaturated fats that we need to keep our skin healthy. They are rich in phyto-chemicals and vitamins that helps slow down the process of ageing by preventing cell damage.

5. Ginger and garlic

These are used in minor quantities in our food but they play a major role in our life. Studies suggest that the component allicin present in them act as anti-inflammatory agents and they also have anti-fungal properties. Garlic also helps in lowering cholesterol, blood pressure, and prevents cell degeneration.

6. Avocado

Avocado is rich in vitamin E that helps in skin repair and reducing blood pressure. It is also rich in folate and hence helps in preventing osteoporosis. Use avocado dip with a slice of bread or salad to get the benefit.

So why not combine these few anti-ageing foods and relish some delicious recipes?

1. Berry Blast

Makes 12 halves

Serving Size: 2 halves

Serves 6

Cooking time: 60 mins

Ingredients

1 litre toned milk (3.5% fat)

Juice of 1 lemon

3 tbsp powdered sugar

6 medium strawberries

Method

1. Boil 1 litre of milk; turn off heat and add lemon juice and let the milk curdle. If it does not curdle, add more lemon juice. Cover for 2 minutes. Strain through a muslin cloth, making sure all the liquid or whey is removed. What remains in the cloth is *paneer.*

2. Churn the *paneer* in a blender for 3 seconds. Combine powder sugar with the churned paneer while it is hot on a flat plate.

3. Mash by hand until a soft dough is formed and sugar is completely dissolved (approximately 5 minutes). Deep freeze for 20 minutes.

4. Divide the mixture into 6 equal parts. Wrap up each part around one strawberry, such that it takes the shape of the strawberry.

5. Refrigerate once again for 30-40 minutes. Slice each piece length-wise into half, with a butter knife. Serve chilled.

Value per serving (2 halves)

Calories 148 kcal

Protein 5 gms

Fat 7 gms

Carbs 16 gms

Calcium 204 mgs

Iron 1 mg

Fibre 0 gm

2. Masala Booster

Makes 3 glasses

Serving Size: 1 glass

Serves 3

Cooking time: 5 mins

Ingredients

1 cup fat-free curd, made from 400 ml fat-free milk (0–0.8% fat)

2 cups water

1 tsp powdered sugar

Salt to taste

½ greenchilli, chopped finely

1/4th inch piece of ginger, chopped finely

1/4th tsp jeera powder (cumin powder)

1/4th tsp jeera (cumin seeds)

1/4th tsp mustard seeds

2 tsp fresh coriander leaves, finely chopped

½ tsp oil

Method

1. Place the curd, water, sugar, salt, green chilli, ginger and cumin powder in a vessel. Churn with a hand blender and strain.
2. Heat oil in a small pan. Add jeera and mustard seeds; once they begin to splutter, add to the prepared buttermilk.
3. Serve in a tall glass. Garnish with coriander.

Value per serving(1 glass)

Calories 36 kcal

Protein 2 gms

Fat 1 gm

Carbs 5 gms

Calcium 89 mgs

Iron 0 mg

Fibre 0 gm

3. *Farmer's Special*

Makes 2 ½ cups

Serving Size: 1 cup

Serves 2

Cooking time: 25 mins

Ingredients

    50 gms mushrooms, chopped coarsely

    100 gms tofu, cubed

    1 small head of broccoli (60 gms), separated into small florets

    1 medium red and yellow bell pepper, cubed

    1 medium onion, cubed

    1 medium tomato, cubed

    4 tbsp ketchup

    ½ tsp red chilli powder

    Salt as per taste

    2 tbsp oil

Method

1. Bring water to boil in a large pan and add broccoli.
2. After 2 minutes add bell peppers followed by mushrooms, and drain.
3. In a separate pan, heat oil; sauté onions until translucent. Add in the boiled vegetables and seasoning (salt and chilli powder); stir-fry for a while.
4. Mix in the tomatoes; let it cook for 2 minutes, then add ketchup. Simmer for about 3 minutes.
5. Add the tofu and cook for another 3–4 minutes. Serve hot.

Value per serving (1 cup)

    Calories 132 kcal

    Protein 8 gms

    Fat 5 gms

    Carbs 15 gms

Calcium 158 mgs

Fibre 2 gms

Iron 0.8 mg

4. *Sweet Bonanza*

Makes 4 cup

Serving Size: ½ cup

Serves 4

Soaking time: 5 hrs

Cooking time: 10 mins

Ingredients

½ of 1 large apple (or any other fruit of your choice)

3 cups fresh curd, made from 1 litre toned milk (3.5% fat; hung for 5 hours)

4 almonds, chopped coarsely

2 tbsp crystallized sugar

2 tbsp powdered sugar

A pinch of cinnamon powder

Method

1. Grease a plate with a drop of *ghee* and set aside.
2. Now make the praline by heating 2 tbsp crystallized sugar in a pan and stir it continuously with a fork, let it melt and caramelize to a golden-brown liquid. Remove from heat and add almonds.
3. Immediately spread the praline mixture on the greased plate.
4. Once set and cooled completely, blend it in a mixer for 2 seconds. Set aside.

5. Make the hung curd by straining the curd through the muslin cloth. Add the cinnamon and powdered sugar.
6. Peel the apple and cut into fine cubes. Add to the curd.
7. Mix in ¾ of the praline. Refrigerate.
8. To serve, pour the fruit cream into 4 small cups and decorate each with the remaining praline. Serve chilled.

Value per serving(1/2 cup)

Calories 180 kcal

Protein 5 gms

Fat 7 gms

Carbs 23 gms

Calcium 253 mgs

Iron 1 mg

Fibre 0 gm

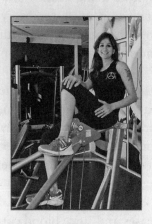

SHALINI BHARGAVA,
FITNESS TRAINER

A common friend introduced me to Shalini. I would always admire her muscle tone whenever I'd meet her, so there was no better person to ask to write about the importance of health and weight training for beauty and skin than her. Very kind of you to keep giving in to all the versions I asked you to write :)

Anti-ageing workout

We all equate exercise and workouts with weight loss and hot sculpted bodies. But do we know that being thin does not always mean being healthy and fit?

Regular exercise is a must for everyone because of cardiovascular health, muscle health, functioning of the body systems and for women, most importantly for the bones and skin.

Along with a healthy diet, lots of water, supplementation, stress management, sun protection, and exercise is an important and integral part of healthy bones and skin and to prevent or delay the early signs of ageing.

Along with the cardiovascular benefits of physical activity, anything that promotes healthy circulation also helps keep your skin healthy and vibrant. During exercise, blood flow increases and since blood carries oxygen and nutrients to all cells of the body, the skin cells also get more nourished. In addition to providing oxygen, blood flow also helps carry away waste products, including free radicals from the cells. Contrary to some claims, exercise doesn't detoxify the skin. The job of neutralizing toxins belongs mostly to the liver. But by increasing blood flow, a bout of exercise helps flush cellular debris out of the system and cleans the skin from inside. Besides the activation of the blood circulatory system, the lymphatic system is also activated which helps faster removal of cellular wastes and toxins.

Exercise also releases the good mood hormones, particularly the endorphins, which help release stress. And by decreasing stress, some conditions like acne and eczema can be reduced.

Regular exercise helps tone muscles and firmer muscles definitely help the skin look tighter and younger, making you look better overall.

Besides the above, regular exercise is very important for our bones and muscle strength too.

Like muscle, bone is living tissue that responds to exercise by becoming stronger. Regular exercise helps achieve greater peak bone mass (maximum bone density and strength). For most people, bone mass peaks during the 30s. After that, we begin to lose bone. Women and men older than age 20 can help prevent bone loss with regular exercise. Exercising allows us to maintain muscle strength, coordination, and balance, which in turn helps to prevent falls and related fractures. This is especially important for older adults and people who have been diagnosed with osteoporosis.

The best bone-building exercises

The best exercise for your bones is the weight-bearing kind, which forces you to work against gravity. Some examples of weight-bearing exercises include weight training, walking, hiking, jogging, climbing stairs, tennis, and dancing. Examples of exercises that are not weight-bearing include swimming and bicycling. Although these activities help build and maintain strong muscles and have excellent cardiovascular benefits, they are not the best way to exercise your bones.

Some modes of exercises which are effective and fun and are the latest fitness trends are:

Yoga

Yoga tops the charts when it comes to a well-rounded exercise modality. Yoga practice helps develop the body and mind bringing a lot of health benefits like:

- Improved blood and Lymphatic circulation
- A light, supple body
- A body that remains alert and active
- Strong bones and muscle
- Fat reduction
- Increased physical strength
- Improved appetite
- Increased capability of coping with fatigue and stress

Yoga has the potential to reduce facial wrinkles and produce a natural 'face-lift'. This is mainly due to the inverted postures such as the head and handstands.

Doing these postures for a few minutes each day has the potential to reverse the effect of gravity and use it to our advantage.

It also increases the circulation to the face that brings much needed nutrients and oxygen to rejuvenate and remove toxin causing matter. Mentally you will become calmer and your body will not experience stress like effects that will cause you to frown and screw up your face.

Also you will sleep a lot better and this always helps in a fresh ready to go look.

The result is firmer facial muscles, which cause a reduction in wrinkles, and a natural face-lift.

The inverted yoga postures often delay the onset of gray hair or hair fall. This is due to the inverted postures causing an increase in blood supply to the hair follicles in the scalp.

Increased flexibility of the neck produced by the asanas also helps by removing the pressure on the blood vessels and nerves in the neck, therefore giving the head an even greater blood supply to the scalp.

The nerves in the neck supply the scalp muscles and the release of pressure on the nerves in the neck will help the scalp muscles to relax.

Some postures are:

Adho Mukho Svanasana: The downward facing dog pose strengthens the arms and shoulders, increases circulation to the head and face, stimulates the nerves of the scalp, tones the muscles and rejuvenates the body.

Steps to do this pose: Lie on your stomach on your yoga mat. Now, place your palms near your ears and point your toes downwards so that your heels are facing the ceiling. Now exhale and push off your hands such that your buttocks point towards the sky. In this pose you will look like an inverted 'V'. Now push back onto your feet so that they are flat on the floor. You will feel a stretch on your hamstrings. Do not walk closer to your hands to put your feet flat on the floor, this defeats the purpose of doing this pose. Practice this regularly and you will slowly increase your flexibility and be able to flatten your feet.

Uttanasana: This is a forward-bending pose that stretches out the hamstrings, and the muscles of the abdomen. It also makes the blood rush to your head, helping your body switch from the sympathetic to the parasympathetic nervous system, helping you relax.

Steps to do this pose: To perform this pose, stand straight. Raise your hands from the front to above your head as you inhale slowly. Then bend forward completely pushing your buttocks back till your palms touch the floor and your forehead touches your knees. If you cannot bend completely, or are uncomfortable with the stretch on your hamstrings, bend your knees a little. Stay in this pose till you are comfortable. To return back to the standing position, as you inhale slowly bring your arms above your head, raising your upper body. Then as you exhale bring your arms down from front of your face. Do not jerk up. Remember to rise up from the hips, without straining your muscles.

Vajrasana: This is a simple pose that is great to relax the mind and improve digestion. It is believed that a good digestive system is the key to a healthy body. Therefore this asana is ideal to improve hair growth. Vajrasana also massages the kanda spot about 12 inches above the anus that is the point of convergence of over 72,000 nerves.

Steps to do this pose: All you need to do is place a yoga mat on the floor. Kneel on the mat, and let the top surface of your feet touch the mat such that your heels are pointing upwards. Now gently place your buttocks on your heels. It is important to note that your heels are on either side of your anus. Now place both your palms on your knees, facing downwards. Close your eyes and breathe in deeply at a steady rate.

Pawanmuktasana/Apanasana: This asana helps relieve any gas built up in the stomach and abdomen and assists in better digestion, thereby purifying the blood and improving the growth of hair by stimulating hair follicles. Apanasana is also a great pose for relaxing the back and the tense muscles of the neck and thighs.

Steps to do this pose: Lie on your back, and place your palms on your knees. As you exhale pull your legs to your chest gently. Allow your legs to move with the strength of your thighs rather than using your arms to pull them in too much. When you inhale loosen your grip, allowing your legs to move completely away from your tummy. Do this for a few breaths at your own pace. Let your breath guide your movement. Hold this position for some time. Close your eyes, and if your mind is not at rest, try counting your breaths. This helps you calm down. When you feel calm, slowly lower your legs to the floor and relax.

Sarvangasana: This pose is essentially known for its ability to regulate the working of the thyroid glands and helps the head get ample supply of blood, helping in hair growth. Since the thyroid glands are responsible for the proper functioning of the entire body including the digestive, nervous and reproductive systems, regulating metabolism and the working of the respiratory system and mitigating hair fall, this pose is a boon for those suffering from conditions like male pattern baldness, female pattern baldness, and hair fall due to hormonal imbalance. Apart from that, it nourishes the spine with a good supply of blood and oxygen, helping you beat nervous system disorders, and improving your all round health.

Steps to do this pose: Lie on a yoga mat with your legs extending outwards. Now slowly raise your legs either by first folding them at the knees or by lifting them straight. Place your palms along your back and hips to support it, and raise your body while pointing your toes to the ceiling. All your weight should be on your shoulders. Make sure you breathe slowly and lock your chin into your chest. Your elbows should be touching the floor and your back should be supported. Hold this pose for as long as you are comfortable. To return to the lying position, slowly lower your body. Do not fall back to the lying position.

Tips to keep in mind: Do not do this pose if you suffer from any neck or spinal injuries. If you do have high blood pressure, perform this exercise only under supervision.

High intensity interval training

High-intensity interval training (HIIT), also called High-Intensity Intermittent Exercise (HIIE) or sprint interval training (SIT), is an enhanced form of interval training, an exercise strategy alternating periods of short intense anaerobic exercise with less-intense recovery periods. HIIT is a form of cardiovascular exercise. Usual HIIT sessions may vary from 4–30 minutes. These short, intense workouts provide improved athletic capacity and condition, improved glucose metabolism, and improved fat burning.

Dance fitness workouts

Masala bhangra: The Masala Bhangra Workout is an exercise dance routine that modernizes the high-energy folk dance of Bhangra by blending traditional Bhangra dance steps and the exhilaration of Bollywood (Hindi film) moves. This unique dance mixes cardiovascular with fun, and is suitable for participants of all ages and fitness levels.

Zumba: Zumba involves dance and aerobic elements. Zumba's music and choreography incorporates hip-hop, soca, samba, salsa, merengue, mambo, bhangra, martial arts, and some Bollywood and belly dance moves.

Piloxing

The program uniquely blends the power, speed, and agility of boxing with the targeted sculpting and flexibility of pilates. These techniques are also supplemented by the use of weighted gloves, further toning the arms and maximizing cardiovascular health. Add to that exhilarating dance moves and you have a muscle-toning, fat-burning workout that will make you feel physically and mentally empowered!

Necessary tip:

If you have health problems—such as heart trouble, high blood pressure, diabetes, or obesity—or if you are 40 or older, check with your doctor before you begin a regular exercise programme.

Listen to your body. When starting an exercise routine, you may have some muscle soreness and discomfort at the beginning, but this should not be painful or last more than 48 hours. If it does, you may be working too hard and need to ease up. Stop exercising if you have any chest pain or discomfort, and see your doctor before your next exercise session.

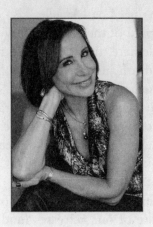

DR AVA SHAMBAN, MD
CELEBRITY DERMATOLOGIST

I first met Ava at the annual meeting of the American Society for Dermatologic Surgery (ASDS) in Chicago where I was the only Indian faculty member who was invited. Amid a very warm and welcoming group of doctors, I find a soft spoken, almost shy lady with a childlike smile. I connected with her that very minute. Later I invited her to one of my sessions at the Anti-ageing Medicine World Congress in Monte-Carlo. Before introducing her to the audience, I looked her up on the Internet and found out just how popular she was—a celebrity dermatologist no less! So there you go—I bring you the very best from the West as well.

Red Carpet Ready, 24/7

My hometown in Los Angeles is considered the rejuvenation capital of the world and with good reason. For many people here, their looks is a matter of career life and career death just as it is in Bollywood. Today, with our entrenched celebrity culture, ultra-exposure 24/7, and invasive 'gotcha' paparazzi practices, the stars are not only photographed on the red carpet but whilst dropping off their kids on the school run too. And the pressure to look amazing even in the most casual or intimate settings is daunting.

This means that we in the rejuvenation business have to take extra care of our actresses (and actors) so that they can enjoy their treatments in private—and the results in public—without punishing media commentary. Believe me, for all the press deconstruction of who has done what and when, I can tell you that there are ten times as many celebrities whose faces and bodies escape this scrutiny because their improvements are done so skillfully and look so natural. And the good news is that the celebrity treatments are available for you.

While getting older is inevitable, looking older is totally negotiable with preventative home care playing a huge part in keeping time off your face (and body, and hands).

Hollywood is all about getting optimal results on an accelerated timeframe. Whether you are walking the red carpet or preparing for a date or job interview, the same principles apply to designing your routine.

I am going to outline several different skin scenarios most commonly seen in Hollwood:

How to look good post having a baby

Confidence and lots of it! I see many women (especially in L.A) who are insecure with their post baby bodies and their skin. Some have melasma and dark circles. Stop stressing about it. You just created life. Most can be fixed and corrected with peels, skincare, and lasers. Get monthly facials and be consistent with your skincare routine to regain your pregnancy glow.

How to look fresh after a fierce workout

In Hollywood, fitness is more important than ever. Fitness=getting sweaty and burning calories. It's not a beauty pageant, so no thick foundation at the gym. It can clog your pores and lead to breakouts after a sweaty workout. In your gym bag, pack some salicylic acid pads that you can use to quickly wipe off your skin. Always have a travel size sunscreen to apply immediately after the wipes. Twist your hair into a fishtail braid, apply mascara and lip gloss.

How to look stunning before a last minute date night

Now with both texting and dating apps, your next date may be only ten minutes away. Fresh glowing skin is the first sign of beauty. A nice shortcut is to do five minutes of exercise that will bring blood to your face such as a series of yoga poses or high-intensity dancing. Run an ice cube over your face followed by application of natural oil such as grape seed oil or coconut oil. It will make your skin soft and glowing, perfectly prepared for a light application of make up or just glow and go.

How to make your lips look kissable

Exfoliating the lips may sound strange but is an effective starting point to softer lips. You can make a lip scrub yourself or look for one that has granular sugar. Don't go overboard. You don't want your lips raw and bleeding but a gently exfoliation can make them both smooth and a little more plump. After exfoliation, make sure to apply a moisturizing lip balm containing SPF. If your lips need an extra pout, you may want to visit your doctor's office to have hyaluronic acid injections to complete your juicy pout. Research supports the popular concept that men are more drawn to a woman's pout over any other facial feature.

How to get Red Carpet Ready: At-home approach

How you care for your skin at home is every bit as important as what we do in the office. To minimize ageing, in addition to daily sunscreen devotion, good sense and good health are what your skin needs to stay both looking and actually functioning younger. Eat lots of fruits and vegetables, avoid junk food, exercise regularly and get plenty of rest. By day, you'll want to use topical sun protection and antioxidants on all the exposed areas. By night a retinol, peptide, or growth factor should be applied to the face, neck, and chest.

Here are my guidelines to achieve that celebrity glow even beyond award season:

Get a skincare regimen, and stick with it

IN THE MORNING:

> **Step 1)** Cleanse
>
> **Step 2)** Moisturize and add antioxidants
>
> **Step 3)** Protect (Use SPF of at least 30 everyday)

EVENING:

> **Step 1)** Cleanse with a gentle exfoliator such as salicylic acid or an ultrasound cleansing brush
>
> **Step 2)** Nourish with peptides
>
> **Step 3)** Moisturize

*Don't forget to switch your products every season. In the warmer months, a lighter moisturizer will suffice. In the colder months, a heavier moisturizer will be needed.

My favourite D.I.Y Recipes

Eating green and clean is the way of living out here in Los Angeles. Organic food as well as organic skincare is also very popular. So in order to get truly organic ingredients, you have to make it yourself.

Oily Skin:

- **Papaya Lemon Cleanser**
  ½ papaya, 2 tbsp witch hazel, 1 tsp lemon juice
  Mix ingredients, use with washcloth, rinse with warm water.
- **Pomegranate Toner**
  2 tbsp pomegranate juice, 1 tbsp witch hazel, 2 tsp vodka, ½ tsp sea salt

Combine all ingredients and shake well. Use a cotton pad to apply to the face.

Normal Skin:

❖ **Blueberry Mask**
½ cup blueberries, 1 tbsp rice flour, 2 tbsp yogurt
Place the blueberries in a glass bowl and smash them with a fork. Add other ingredients and mix well. Spread on your face, neck, and chest. Leave on for fifteen minutes. Rinse off with warm water.

❖ **Calendula and Chamomile Cream**
½ cup bland face cream, 1 tbsp almond oil, 1 tsp calendula extract, 5 drops calendula oil, 5 drops chamomile oil
Use day or night.

Dry Skin:

❖ **Milk Mask**
2 tbsp powdered milk, ¼ cup yogurt, ½ tsp honey
Mix all ingredients and apply to face and neck for 15 minutes. Rinse with room temperature water.

❖ **Sweet and Good Yogurt Scrub**
1 egg white, ½ cup yogurt, 2 tbs brown sugar
Beat egg white, add yogurt and sugar. Gently scrub your face with the mixture, and then rinse with warm water.

How to get Red Carpet Ready: With in-office techniques and technologies

These are some of the newest technologies available in the dermatological world today. Keep in mind downtime and visible results vary. So if you have a big event, make sure to schedule the procedures in an appropriate manner. In the office, we like to use a multimodal approach to enhance results.

- ❖ Skin Tightening
- ❖ Facial Volume
- ❖ Fine Lines and Wrinkles
- ❖ Skin Retexturing
- ❖ Laser Hair Removal
- ❖ Skin Resurfacing

And finally, in my professional opinion, having a good laugh with people you love can erase years from your face because it makes everyone look totally alive and absolutely beautiful.

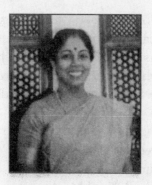

ARUNDHATHI RAI,
NATUROPATH

She's the naturopath we've been referring to in the book. Now it's time for the big reveal! She's none other than my beautiful Mangalorean mumma! Right from when we were young, she taught me to admire beauty and to do every little thing beautifully—whether it was dressing up or setting a table or arranging the wardrobe. I even got an award in school because my teacher could never find a single crease on my uniform throughout the year! That's my mom for you—perfect to the tee. Home care is so imbibed in me because of her—she has a remedy in her kitchen for every little thing. Thank you mom for not only making me a doctor but encouraging me to be an all-rounder. Love you much.

Home remedies for beautiful skin

Sugar in honey: A moisturizing scrub that brings back the shine. Splash some warm water on your face and then on wet, clean face, apply honey and sugar mixed together. Using your fingertips very gently massage all over with circular motion. Wash off with water. See your skin glow.

Yogurt **and strawberry:** Mash a few strawberries into yogurt. Apply all over your face and neck. Gently massage; the tiny seeds that you see on the strawberry peels acts as a scrub. Let it sit for about 10 minutes. Wash off with tap water.

Banana: Got banana that have gone too ripe? Don't dunk them in the trash, instead mash them and apply on your face and hands. Wash off after about 10 minutes. Your skin will be super soft and moisturized.

Papaya: Papaya has an enzyme called papain which can removes the dead skin cells and makes the skin very firm. Mash a few pieces of papaya and apply all over your face and neck. Keep on for 10 to 15 minutes. Wash off with slightly warm water. Your skin feels supple and dewy.

Neem: Once I had met the head of an international skincare brand who was talking to me about this great new product they were coming up with—neem. Hello! We have known about it since ages. Neem is a cure-all for any form of skin infection or trouble. It is a very good antiseptic. Neem can be drunk as shots, applied as paste on the face, or used as a gentle scrub in its raw form. It is great for acne prone skin.

Sandalwood paste: Make a paste by rubbing it on a rough stone with rose water or milk as a medium. You can refrigerate it for a week or more. Just apply a layer of it every day. It makes your skin flawless. It takes care of pigmentation and dull skin beautifully.

Lemon: Yes, the magic ingredient from the kitchen. I am sure all of us have access to this one. Great on acne prone skin, opens up pores, and oily skin. Just over turn half a lemon and apply all over the area that looks tanned. The citric acid in it lightens pigmentation effectively. You can use lemon to take care of yellow nails too. Great as a regular skin lightening cleanser, when you mix the juice of a lemon with besan (gramflour) and use that to wash your face. When used in the last rinse during hair wash, it leaves hair with a glam shine.

Coconut milk: Skin feeling dull and dehydrated? Then extract milk from the grated pulp of a coconut. Apply all over your face and hands. Wash off after a while. Skin will feel soft and nourished.

Tender coconut water: If your skin is feeling grimy and taut, then applying tender coconut water directly to your skin will cleanse and remove any excess oil/dirt. It will instantly hydrate your skin thoroughly.

Apple cider vinegar: Mix some apple cider vinegar with little water and soak a piece of muslin in it. Apply over your face and lie down to relax. Take off after the vinegar dries up on your face. Then rinse with cold water. Your skin will look radiant. It is great for dealing with pigmentation. A naturopath once told me, 2 spoons of apple cider vinegar in warm water before bed time is the thing to do.

Rosewater and milk: Back from the sun with burning red skin? Mix some chilled milk with rosewater and apply on the affected areas. Leave on for few minutes, and wash off with cold water. Skin will be soothed and calmed instantly. The lactic acid in milk also fights tan from settling on the skin.

Cucumber and potato pack: Want to rejuvenate patchy skin and dark under eye area? Then grate half a cucumber and potato and apply all over face, neck and even hands. Keep on for 15 minutes or so and then rinse

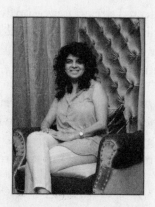

DR ANJALI CHHABRIA,
CONSULTANT AND PSYCHIATRIST

She's a senior doctor whom I'd occasionally meet at common forums where we'd be called in as experts. She has always been a very loving and encouraging senior. Each time I hear her speak, it makes me wiser emotionally. It's her smile and warmth that touches me the most.

Impact of ageing on a woman's mind

Picture this: A room full of people sitting and chatting away, and suddenly all their heads turn at once to a woman walking in, her head held high, a walk of elegance and poise. Every eye is on her, admiring her sheer beauty and grace. Which woman does not want this? For many women, feeling good about oneself has a lot to do with looking good and getting compliments for the same.

As Indian women, if we were to look at the majority, we'd find that many women nowadays are making an effort to look good much more than before. Women today are more financially independent, and therefore are more adept at making their own decisions of choosing to indulge themselves. Also, advancements in beauty products have further simplified the process.

Beauty is a term that has been closely associated with women for centuries. It is best depicted by women as they are the more aesthetically pleasing sex of the two. This does not necessarily mean that for women looking good is a 'passport' to a great life, but it definitely is of core importance for self-acceptance and confidence. In a society preoccupied with outward appearances, women place beauty near the top of their priority list. Dealing with change in appearance is an inevitable process. Women deal with acne at puberty to pigmentation and wrinkles at menopause when they are 60....phew! From a young age, measures are taken to maintain a certain standard of beauty. High heels, crash diets, painful beautifying procedures, women do it all to make heads turn. The benefits of looking good are not just attention and appreciation by others, but also achieving self-confidence and sense of worth.

Changes in appearance are more pronounced as a woman ages. Wrinkles, crow's feet, under-eye bags, graying and thinning hair...the list is endless. Different women have varying perceptions of ageing. For some women, ageing is akin to 'losing all the wealth' they had. Visible signs of ageing cannot be avoided or controlled, and so some may feel they are losing control over a significant part of their lives. There are also women who are least concerned about ageing and its effects. They are very comfortable with grey hair and that extra tire around their waists. Some women are so confident and comfortable with themselves that they automatically age gracefully. They believe in wholeheartedly embracing the change instead of rectifying them. These women may be more independent mentally, free from society pressures. They may not feel the need for any reassurance from others. With the changes in society, women are increasingly becoming career-oriented and independent. Their sense of self is derived from their career, education, achievements, etc. whereas aesthetics are given lesser importance. On the other hand, women who lead a mundane life as housewives are so bogged down by domestic responsibilities, that they do not find the energy or time to indulge in cosmetic procedures despite having the inclination.

A majority of women have been found to be apprehensive about their looks. To add to it, changes in appearance come with no prior notice. In an attempt to immortalize their youth, one will find that women would rather be addressed by their first names as opposed to the traditional term: 'Aunty'. Some women resist change and some welcome it. It depends on personality and coping mechanisms of a woman.

So to what extent does one go or where must one go to make oneself feel 'stunning'. Do you constantly wait to see the first white strand of hair before you want to colour it again or do you just walk out of the house, grey hair and all?

Well, how much should one invest in one's looks is a personal choice. But looking good does go a long way with self-confidence. If investing a little into 'feeling special' makes you feel good and fit about yourself, go ahead and indulge. But it has to be a personal choice. It cannot be imposed nor should it be a competition with one's peers. If I was to go a step further, looking good is not just external but internal as well. Besides taking care of your outward appearance, it is also important to feel good emotionally. Doing activities which make you feel good, socializing, being emotionally and physically active helps to attain a feeling of empowerment.

When you look at yourself in the mirror, you should see a reflection of a good looking person who radiates happiness. The attraction quotient increases with your happiness quotient. The happier you are, the more attractive you will feel and therefore, look. So if looking good adds to your happiness, go for it but it shouldn't become a cause of 'distress'. Flaunt your assets and feel good about yourself. You are worth every bit of it.

CONCLUSION

I FIRMLY BELIEVE MY practice has been built over the years only and only by word of mouth since every patient who walked in during the initial days was either a friend or a relative (which is also why confidentiality is top priority in my practice). Recently, we had a big movie star come in for a hair treatment. While my assistant was applying anaesthesia to his scalp, he started chatting up with her. Soon he came to the point and asked, 'Hey what did the other star I referred get done? You can tell me. He is my best buddy.' I am so proud of the way one of my chief staff members handled the situation. She told him, 'Sir, if he is your best buddy, so the right to inform you is his and not mine. To me he is just a client and we strictly abide by the confidentiality rule here.'

Initially when a couple of my patients told me that they got a lot of compliments after my treatments, but when asked, they said it was their new 'yoga routine' because no one could tell what had been changed or done. I used to feel so cheated. All credit due to me was being taken away by some fictitious yoga teacher. Eventually, as I grew in my practice, I realized that beauty and skin and the interventions or efforts towards it was too personal to people as was their deepest emotions. So one may not like to share it with others. And share they did but with their closest ones.

As much as you look good—shape, structurally, and feature wise—if your skin is not looking healthy, youthful, and clear, then nothing is okay. We all know that skin is a reflection of your inner health. Not just skin, your hair and nails are also great markers of your overall health.

In my practice, when I have patients that want to be taken care of or want to enhance something in their appearance, I like to start off with a general set of blood tests—including hormones and nutrient values or maybe an ultrasound of your pelvis—to look at the health of your ovaries. Then I start off with a detailed nutritional plan to get your nutrition at the right levels. If you need hormonal tweaking, then I send you to an endocrinologist to make sure that your health is at its optimum. This is because as you age, your biorhythm, your hormones, and the absorption of various nutrients—all can change. So we start analysing your sleep pattern, your food habits, your nutrition level, your hydration levels etc. to decide the right course of action. My first consultation is my longest and I spend the longest time analysing your face, features, likes, beauty goals, lifestyle, social circle, profession etc.

Then comes in the actual care of skin and hair from the top. So I go over your home care regime—the right sunscreen, the right moisturizer, day cream, and night cream. Along with the oral supplements, you may need to correct your nutrition or your health. Then I move on to making a little skin rejuvenation plan with exfoliating treatments like peels or microdermabrasion. After that, I look at your skin tightening aspects with either lasers or radio frequency. We also take care of pigmentation with specialized lasers or peels if needed. Your skin hydration, health and glow are taken care of with specialized facials.

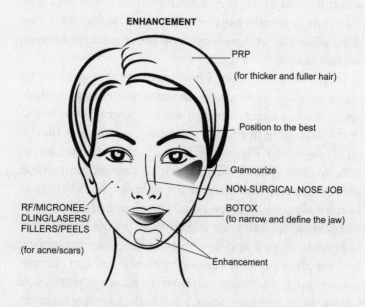

ENHANCEMENT

PRP
(for thicker and fuller hair)

Position to the best

Glamourize

NON-SURGICAL NOSE JOB

BOTOX
(to narrow and define the jaw)

RF/MICRONEE-
DLING/LASERS/
FILLERS/PEELS

(for acne/scars)

Enhancement

Once you finish with this one- or three-month plan, then when your skin starts to look really healthy, we move to taking care of your skin in a slightly more advanced way that deals with your skin collagen and deeper hydration. I treat with maybe PRP or mesotherapy with hyaluronic acid to improve the hydration of the skin, the firmness of the skin, and also the plumpness of your skin. Then I analyse the structure of your face. At times, you may need to dissolve some fat of your jowls, or double chin, or we need to add a bit of volume to areas that have sagged or lift your brows or erase wrinkles with Botox.

While both Aishwarya Rai and Angelina Jolie are individually very good looking women, Angelina's lips on Aishwarya's face would not fit, right? You too need to understand that one feature, one formula, will not fit everyone. I analyse every step to create a customized set of treatments for each of my patients. What I generally do is divide the face into three sections—the upper one third, middle one third, and lower one third. For each section, I analyse the skin, the lines, the volume loss, and the features.

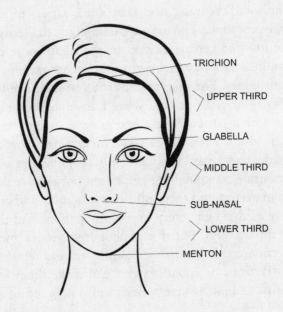

TRICHION

UPPER THIRD

GLABELLA

MIDDLE THIRD

SUB-NASAL

LOWER THIRD

MENTON

Then I see how each of these can be beautified, and how it will impact the look of your whole face. Having said that, I do not work in parts. Imagine trying to do up an expensive vintage car and only doing up the front while neglecting the back—how weird would that look? That is why I take into account the whole of the face and see how little things in each section of the face can be improved to create a beautiful face over all. I also like to work in a progressive manner so that the change is gradual and more natural. I take care of the background issues first like dealing with scars, glow, or pigmentation and then slowly work towards making each feature look good and defined but not artificial.

The first and most important thing, as I mentioned, I do is to evaluate and assess a patient's aesthetic goals and threshold. People come to me for a variety of reasons. It may not always be for a total aesthetic makeover. It may be just for getting advice on the right home care or it could be about acne, pigmentation, or specific skin and hair issues. For such cases, I stick to their need and give them the best options. What I absolutely don't do is to sit with a patient who came in for acne and start telling her how her nose is crooked or that her crow's feet are evident and that I can fix them! I don't believe in drawing attention to something you might not even realize is less than perfect and then leave you miserable and conscious. My goal is help every one of my patient find their own aesthetic bliss. But if a patient were to ask me how to become more beautiful, I go all out and tell them what corrections or enhancements can make them look their absolute best. If that patient walks in wanting me to fix the nose when what they actually need is a fixing of the chin, then I'll guide them towards that.

I like to do it slow and gradual and tell my patients that they should not expect a magic wand to make them look good instantly. Also magic only tends to last for a short moment. I actually work with them for over a month to a year to give them the skin and face that they can really show off. I also understand the importance of no tell-tale signs, so I almost have a zero bruise protocol at our clinic which ensures that my clients can remain worry-free. So patient comfort, their confidentiality, and a natural, almost painless result is what I like to promise my patients.

Change is the only constant. So don't fear the onslaught of the ageing process as it is inevitable. Instead, welcome it using *Age Erase* as your friend, companion, and guide. Here's to ageing gracefully!

ACKNOWLEDGEMENTS

ROME WASN'T BUILT IN a day and this book didn't happen in a day either. It took the time and love of many to make *Age Erase* a reality.

I'd first like to start by thanking all the experts—Anjali Chhabria, Ava Shamban, Ranjana Dhanu, Pooja Makhija, Suman Agarwal, Shalini Bhargava, and Arundhathi Rai—for their invaluable contribution to my book.

To all the stars—Shilpa, Sania, Nargis, Yami, Shruti, Sarika, Akshara, Nagarjuna, Suriya, Rana, Jackky, Dino, Mini, Sandip, Gajra, Manasi, Lakshmi, Chandi, Amla, Tamannaah, Aamir, Adha, Sahil, Sukriti, Shilpi, Upasna, Priya, Samantha, Neetu, Anita and Kavita—thank you for taking out time from your busy schedules and contributing to the book in your own way. It feels very nice to know you feel the way you do about me.

To my friends Gajra and Priyanka Bhattacharya and Dr Pushpa Khurana—who was a resident and associate at my Hyderabad clinic and now has a successful practice in Punjab—for the final edits when my brain shut off and Maneka Hunjan for helping me with the pharmacological gyan in the cosmeceuticals chapter. Thank you Mahindra for the beautiful illustrations. This book wouldn't have been what it is if my friend Milee Ashwarya hadn't pushed me into writing it. So thank you, again!

To my editor Gurveen for giving the book its final shape.

A NOTE ON THE AUTHOR

DR RASHMI SHETTY, INDUSTRY pioneer, celebrity doctor, author, and leading expert in non-surgical aesthetic medicine, graduated from the prestigious Mysore University and holds a Diploma in Cosmetology (Chester, UK), FRSH (UK). Her training in plastic surgery under some of the finest plastic surgeons in the country has been the foundation of her achievements. Her eye for facial aesthetics, excellent injector skills, and her drive to innovate has kept her at the forefront of non-surgical facial aesthetics.

Dr Shetty is renowned internationally in both the academic and industry arenas for her unique knowledge, skills, and abilities and has been a domain expert at International congresses and training courses. She is the only Indian doctor on the international advisory board of the Anti-ageing World Congress. She is also on the scientific advisory board for Aesthetics Asia & 1st Aesthetics and Anti-ageing Medicine Asian Congress (AMAC).

She is the reason behind some of the most beautiful celebrity faces in India and has led launches of many of the largest aesthetic injectable products like Juvederm, Voluma, and Refine. She is also a panel expert for Unilever for skincare, Marico for Hair Care, Allergan for Botox and Juvederm, and forums like Femina Miss India, Actor Prepares etc.

Her vibrant practice includes her private clinic, Ra Skin 'n' Aesthetics in Santa Cruz (Mumbai) and Reva Health & Skin (Hyderabad). She also leads the Aesthetics industry with the ongoing product and technology evaluation and research at her clinic.

You can contact her at:

Website: www.drrashmishetty.com
Twitter: @drrashmishetty
Facebook: www.facebook.com/drrashmiraishetty
Email: ageerase@drrashmishetty.com